Wing Chun

The Ultimate Guide to Starting Wing Chun

(Strengthen Your Wing Chun Skills and Understand the Core Concepts)

George Swift

Published By **Cathy Nedrow**

George Swift

All Rights Reserved

Wing Chun: The Ultimate Guide to Starting Wing Chun (Strengthen Your Wing Chun Skills and Understand the Core Concepts)

ISBN 978-0-9950956-9-4

No part of this guidebook shall be reproduced in any form without permission in writing from the publisher except in the case of brief quotations embodied in critical articles or reviews.

Legal & Disclaimer

The information contained in this book is not designed to replace or take the place of any form of medicine or professional medical advice. The information in this book has been provided for educational & entertainment purposes only.

The information contained in this book has been compiled from sources deemed reliable, and it is accurate to the best of the Author's knowledge; however, the Author cannot guarantee its accuracy and validity and cannot be held liable for any errors or omissions. Changes are periodically made to this book. You must consult your doctor or get professional medical advice before using any of the suggested remedies, techniques, or information in this book.

Upon using the information contained in this book, you agree to hold harmless the Author from and against any damages, costs, and expenses, including any legal fees potentially resulting from the application of any of the information provided by this guide. This disclaimer applies to any damages or injury caused by the use and application, whether directly or indirectly, of any advice or information presented, whether for breach of contract, tort, negligence, personal injury, criminal intent, or under any other cause of action.

You agree to accept all risks of using the information presented inside this book. You need to consult a professional medical practitioner in order to ensure you are both able and healthy enough to participate in this program.

Table Of Contents

Chapter 1: The Difference In Styles 1

Chapter 2: Where Does Wing Chun Come From? 12

Chapter 3: The Momentous Life Of Ip Man 22

Chapter 4: Yin And Yang......................... 32

Chapter 5: Open Palm Strikes 41

Chapter 6: Splitting Hand 54

Chapter 7: The Basics Of Siu Lim Tau 74

Chapter 8: The Basics Of Bie-Gee 85

Chapter 9: Free Hand Techniques 103

Chapter 10: Instructors Belt 118

Chapter 11: Wing Chun? 126

Chapter 12: What Does A Typical Class Consist Of?... 138

Chapter 13: Empty Hand Wing Chun Forms 147

Chapter 14: Wing Chun Techniques 157

Chapter 15: The 3 Non-Negotiable Elements 172

Chapter 1: The Difference In Styles

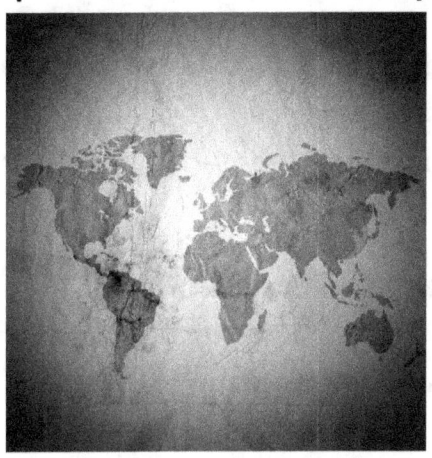

Much like numerous Martial Arts Kung Fu has been adapted across the globe to a variety of distinct styles and organizations.

This variety creates a fascinating and vibrant community of people who all have different viewpoints regarding, what's at the very least, on paper the same form of art. Do you practice the traditional Shaolin techniques? Perhaps you're using one of the five method family techniques such as Lau or the less well-known Mok Gar?

Perhaps you're somewhere between the two, using techniques that are sourced from a variety of types of groups. No matter what your affiliation is, you must A. Accept that there are variations across the globe, and B. Be open to these differences without condemnation.

The main difference between the skilled and knowledgeable martial artist and one who just wants to satisfy their self-interest can be seen in their approach toward other forms of art.

The book also aims at certain styles that is, in this case, the practice that is Wing Chun (Ving Tsun). It would be almost impossible to include all different regional styles around the globe therefore the most popular and general requirements have been in the book when it is it is possible.

The majority of the methods and curriculum included follow the same format, but I can almost swear that there will be some differences, particularly if use a different method in your own club.

However, the fundamentals that is Kung Fu and the many guidelines are common to all and, therefore, even if you aren't a practitioner of Wing Chun you will still get useful info and general guidelines on how to be a successful learner.

Learning through all avenues is crucial in order to be a successful Martial Artist.

The Meaning of 'Kung Fu'

"Kung Fu" is synonymous in western culture with the notion that it is Martial Arts, particularly those that are of Chinese Origin. However, while the concept has at least an accurate geographical location, the definition of the term has changed slightly throughout the years, due to the increasing popularity of the styles has spread across the globe.

Students studying Wing Chun for example are also students of Kung Fu, but practitioners of

Kung Fu do not necessarily take classes in Wing Chun.

The term "Kung Fu often referred to Gung Fu or GongFu originates from China and is an ability that is developed with hard work or by the application of effort or ability to practice and work in order to complete the goal. One reason for the variety of definitions of the word is because, like the majority of Martial Arts terminology the term originated from a distinct language, cannot immediately translate into a unique Western term.

This can be a challenging concept to comprehend when they are studying words that come with multiple or even subtly different meanings.

GMng is a term that can mean the effort, accomplishment or the value of these.

Fk is a man's name in the context of the previous expression.

Most people think the term Kung Fu refers simply to Chinese Martial Arts and while it is true that it can be broadly defined be true, the term "WuShu" is actually more accurate description of this.

However, the term "Kung Fu is now an integral part of Martial Arts vernacular that it is now perfectly normal to refer to it in this manner. So, you can describe your martial arts training by the name of Wing Chun Kung Fu (The Art of) (The Art). Be aware of this when a teacher asks your knowledge of the technical aspect of these, it's important to know what the distinction is.

The Meaning Behind 'Wing-Chun'

The literal translation for Wing-Chun is "yong Chkn" that can translate as "spring Chant". Some practitioners have become a part of the essence that is "Eternal the Springtime". There's a lot of variation regarding how the concept is interpreted by the diverse generation of students who were taught the Wing-Chun instructions from different regions and continents. The fundamental message, however, remains the identical. Most organizations' accepted interpretations vary between "beautiful springtime", "forever springtime" as well as "praising the springtime". Whichever concept, it is an ideal representation of the springtime season. This interpretation could have influenced being the Plum Blossom logo which is now synonymous with the art of Wing-Chun all over the world.

A different theory suggests that the image of popular culture originates from the person who created the martial arts system. The genesis of Wing-Chun as a form of art is usually attributed to a person by the name Ng Mui (see for more details later). This name, no surprise can be translated as "plum bloom". Another explanation is that the plum flower symbolizes the human body. The connection lies in the five points that are now used to represent the head, the two arms and two legs of the human being. This is in accordance in the idea that Wing-Chun may have been the first method to develop its movement based on natural human behavior, rather than from supernatural creatures such as dragons and spirits.

The Wing-Chun (Kung Fu) Salute

Every Martial Arts system has its unique way of how people greet each other. The bow is a popular gesture for both Korean as well as Japanese practice, and the hand salutes used in Kung Fu and Wing-Chun constitute the same method of showing respect. When it comes to Wing-Chun Hand-Clothing, these special hand gestures are traced through the oldest militants. The gestures were used initially to conceal one's identity as belonging to the circle of inner circles.

The most well-known salutation is left palm/right hand. It is actually utilized by a variety of Kung Fu styles. Because of the different translations over time this signal has two distinct meanings. You must consider Kung Fu's Shaolin roots for the primary version.

The fabled Shaolin monks saw their White Tiger and Green Dragon as two animals that had opposing spirit. Therefore, it is natural that the salute used by Kung Fu brings together the White Tiger as well as the Green Dragon with the joining of left and right hands, respectively.

Green Dragon also traditionally symbolizes the direction of east and the season of spring According to Feng Shui. Chinese philosophical thought has classified the dragon as Yang as a male power. Dragons are a symbol of power, resolve, strength, endurance and courage. The dragon guards the divine homes of Gods and Goddesses.

In many ways, the White Tiger exists in sheer contrast in many ways to that of the Green Dragon. So, they be in harmony, and create equilibrium. It is believed that the White Tiger is the symbol of Yin or feminine force because of its inactive nature. It is found in the west, and is a fan of the beauty of autumn. It is portrayed as an armed guard against hostile forces. According to the most ancient Chinese tales that the Green Dragon and White Tiger when they were together, produced the apex of Chi. Like in the Yin and Yang concepts, this pair will never break up.

When performing the Wing-Chun salute, the point of contact of the left hand that is open faces the right-handed fist with care at the centerline. Then they gently shift to the left as they execute an appropriate bow.

The traditional Wing-Chun greeting is done with the hands in opposing places. Hands held in the right position wide while the left hand was clenched into the shape of a fist. The reason for this alteration lies in the third theory. If performed in an ancient reverse-manner salute, it subtly points at the hidden society that created the salute. This can also be referred to as"the "Sun Fist" while the hands that are open is a resemblance to"Crescent Moon" "Crescent moon".

When used in the traditional hand postures that the fist is a representation of the Sun or

Yat and the open hand calls Yuet or the Sun. Moon as well as Yuet. If they are joined, they form one symbol representing the word "bright" and is said similarly to "Ming". It is also interesting that Ming can also be the name of the last Han Dynasty which was deposed by the Manchurians. The group later would create what's now called"the "Ching Dynasty". Ching or Qing refers to the promises of a pure and clear rule. Although this is a date that dates the birth of Wing-Chun in his "Fan Chin Fong Ming", (Overturn the Ching restore the Ming) period, at the time it started to grow it was altered. The fist and palm salute became synonymous with "Return to the Ming".

In the absence of a secret alliance to hide it, this greeting is used as a symbol of respect toward the way of Wing-Chun and the founders, teachers as well as all the people who have been instrumental in its continuing existence. The students in the class learn to express respect to their master, also known as Si-Fu by using this unique salutation. The students are required to practice salutes with the half bow pointed towards the Si-Fu during the beginning and at the end of each class. They are also required to exchange greetings between themselves as they pair up to practice every skill.

The masters of the past faced any adversity they faced so that they could continue to teach the lessons that were taught by Wing-Chun Kuen or "Wing-Chun Fist" And it's that they are worthy of the respect of. Martial artists of today are taught to honor their mentors since they are a source of an abundance of knowledge and data.

Chapter 2: Where Does Wing Chun Come From?

The birth of Wing-Chun is usually attributed to a woman referred to by the name Miss Yim Wing-Chun. Her birthplace was from China and was from Canton, the provincial capital of Canton. Her biography states that she developed into a smart, intelligent morally ethical, and physically fit. In the time that Emperor K'anghsi ruled the throne (between 1662-1722) she was a promise to an individual by the name from Leung Bok Chau. In the time Leung earned his money as a salt merchant in Fukein. In the wake of the loss of her father, Leung discovered her family was in turmoil. Yim Wing-Chun's father man by the name of Yim Yee, was deemed the suspected perpetrator of crime and was imprisoned. The result was that they were obliged to leave. The new house they chose was near the bottom of Tai Leung Mountain, located at the point at the point where Yunnan and Szechaun meet.

It was at this time Kung-Fu was just beginning to take off throughout The Siu Lam Monastery in Honan. It is possible that you are acquainted with the area as it was the location of the well-known Shaolin Temple located on top of Mount Sung. The rate that the system of fighting was advancing was no secret to the prevailing Manchu Command. The previous administration had asked that monks contribute their expertise to the military, but they were refused. In the end, the temple was frequently assaulted. The well-developed martial arts methods gave monks to defend themselves effectively.

In the meantime, a man named Man Wai was completing his Civil Service training. His exam scores were higher than the scores of his fellow students. In an effort to get closer to the administration, he suggested the idea of an unsavory monk under Ma Ning Yee. The aim was to stealthily penetrate and eliminate Siu Lam. Siu Lam. The accomplice of the thief was able discover the blueprints of the temple. The thief was also clever enough to start a chain of fires in the structure. The fires were used as a deterrent and left the monks in danger when soldiers prepared towards a massive attack. In the ensuing battle, several monks were killed.

It was fortunate that the monks who did make it through were suffused with devotion as well as influence. These monks are known today by the Venerable five. They comprised two abbots (Chi-Shin as well as Pak-Mei) Master Mui-Hin, Fung To Tak then the Abbess, Ng-Mui. They managed to find the secret passages and then eluded across the country.

While the four other members of the group began in their pursuit to overthrow the authorities, Ng Mui took a different route. She traveled the country on foot to find the refuge. It was found within the White Crane Temple located on the famous Mount Tae-Leung. The temple was a warm welcome for her and she was granted the opportunity to further her skills. As well as being the top boxer in the country as well, she was also able to find time to research the methods that the army of the state were taught. With careful study, Ng Mui found many faults including their fervent dedication to animalistic designs.

Although they were entertaining however, the styles were not realistic in applications. Actually, a genuine combat between a snake and the snake demonstrated to Ng Mui the manner that each used the other's weakness. The crane was able to block the snake's wings, while invading its beak. However, the snake's approach was direct and clear. Ng Mui was soon to compile the lessons she learned to create a brand new defense strategy.

In the course of her time in the White Crane Temple that Ng Mui travelled to an nearby villages to find bean curd. It was fate that it happened the stand she went to seek out was owned by no other than Yim Yee as well as his daughter. Both women formed an instant bond, one that was soon to prove beneficial to both sides. According to many stories,

Wing-Chun had been accused of being beautiful over the top. In the process, she accidentally was noticed by some of village's most pleasant citizens who tried to force her into marriage. In the wake of learning about her new acquaintance's awkward situation, Ng determined to introduce her brand new technique to Wing-Chun.

To further defend Wing-Chun, she signed a deal with the violent partner. Ng Mui agreed to exile her companion from the village for a period of one year. In this time she was to train her to become a skilled fighter. After a year, they'd be back in order that Wing-Chun as well as her lover could engage in an honest fight. If the guy won, all would be in agreement to the wedding. In the end, Wing-Chun came back after a mere one year. She effortlessly defeated both her adversaries and the posse. She was then granted the right to marry Leung Bok Chau.

The mission was completed, and Ng Mui went home, however, she did not leave without instructing Wing-Chun that she must adhere to her Kung Fu teachings which she was taught. In return, she was instructed to train to someday helping with demolishment of the Manchu administration so to ensure that it could be dissolved and the Ming Dynasty may be restored.

The Ng Mui Legacy

Similar to other martial art philosophies, Wing-Chun Kung Fu has been handed down over many generations. Just as tales and traditions are passed through multiple hands, with minor changes with each passing and crossing, Wing-Chun has also developed. As a result in time and distance, it's difficult to pinpoint the exact route that this method has followed, from its beginning to its current form.

There is a belief that the founder, Yim Wing-Chun, learned the genesis of Wing-Chun through Ng Mui. The evidence for this is evident in the popular Wing-Chun logos. They typically depict the image of a plum blossom.

In Vietnamese the word "Mui" is a reference to the "Mai" flowers. A English version for "Mai" is evidently the plum flower.

One person widely recognized for his role in Kung Fu includes Grandmaster Ip Man. He passed away in the year 1972, however it was not without leaving an important impact on the history of Kung Fu. His methods are a major influence on the ways that Wing-Chun is taught today. Because of the people were his inspirations the practice of Wing-Chun continues to be active and flourishing.

Grandmaster Ip Chun, another renowned person and the his successor to Ip Man is continuing the tradition with greater than just enthusiasm for the Wing-Chun methods. The son of his elder brother continues to promote the art across the globe. The most well-known of his students master is Samuel Kwok. In the present, he is the principal overseas representative for Ip Chun Martial Arts Association. Due to his dedication and hard work to his numerous students and followers, the Wing-Chun tradition is now one of the top martial art forms.

The Ng Mui legacy remains alive to this day by having representatives from that Wing-Chun style passing on their remarkable wisdom to the next generation, and making sure the principles of the traditional Kung Fu never die.

Bruce Lee: The Little Dragon

The most well-known martial actor of all time is without doubt Bruce Lee. Lee's dedication to training brought him the attention of filmmakers of the time created the cult films that we still enjoy today. This is how Lee was as the most well-known name in the world of martial art. Apart from numerous reels of film, you'll also see him mentioned in books, lectures sites, as well as the Bruce Lee foundation. Bruce Lee foundation.

Before becoming an iconic figure, Bruce Lee lived an intriguing life. Bruce Lee was born on November 27 in the year 1940, which was also which was the year that the dragon ruled in the city of San Francisco. Then, shortly afterward they returned home back to Hong Kong. In Hong Kong, his childhood was affected by the turbulent Japanese occupation from 1945 to the present. His first appearance in film occurred as a character in The Beginning of a Boy in the year he turned seven years old. When he was 18, he been in minor parts in a minimum of twenty films. At this time He enrolled at the University of Washington where he was to study philosophical studies.

A constant devotee to Kung Fu, Bruce Lee took some time doing Wing-Chun. He soon realized his style was no longer suitable for him which is why he quit right after acquiring Chum-Kiu. But he was able to adopt Wing-Chun's ideas about energy, speed and relaxation, and incorporate the concepts to his own. This popular method is now called Jeet Kung Do.

The 1960's were when his film-star qualities really caught the attention of audiences when he released The Green Hornet Series. The legacy of his work was further consolidated by the fact that Hong Kong officially backed the creation of his own martial arts films. It is possible to recognize a number of his films because they've since been iconic, highly regarded by fans of martial arts. The collection includes such acclaimed pieces like Fist of Fury, (The Chinese Connection), Enter the Dragon and Return of the Dragon.

These achievements could have been much longer were Bruce Lee not met an tragically early death from Oedema in the old age of just 32. The time Lee was living in Hong Kong working on a film. It could be said that he passed away doing the thing he was most passionate about. Alongside his impressive heritage of martial arts He also leaves behind his spouse Linda along with his daughter Shannon and son Brandon. Brandon along with their child Shannon. However, Brandon would later lose his own life in the filming of The Crow in 1993.

Chapter 3: The Momentous Life Of Ip Man

Ip Man, also referred to as Yip Man, is widely regarded as the great-grandfather of Wing-Chun. The legend of his work is immortalized through film and print. his legacy continues to be felt today.

The birth date was 14 October on the 14th of October in 1893. His life was filled with dramatic events, not the last of which was the instructing a pupil by Bruce Lee. Bruce Lee.

1899 1905 (Ages 6-12)

In his early years living in Foshan, Ip Man was taught Wing-Chun Kung-fu under Chan Wah Shun. The majority of the lessons they occurred at the family's house, located in the main street, or Song Yuen Dai Gai. His peers at time time included Ng Chung So, Ng Siu Lo, Lui Yui Chai and Chan Yui Min.

1905 (Age 12)

Sadly, the great instructor of Ip's Chan Wah Shun passed away and his family in his wake asked for Ng Chung So continue training Ip

Man. Chan Wah Shun's students walked the body of his teacher to Shunde where it was laid to rest.

1905 1907 (Ages 12-14) (Foshan)

As per his master's final wishes, Ip attended training at Ng Chung So's college in Sin Heung Street in the city of Foshan.

1908 (Age 15)

Pong Wai Ting part of Ip Man's family helped him gain the capability to study at St. Stephen College in Hong Kong. At that time Pong Wai Ting lived in a residence located on Craine Road within Hong Kong Island.

1909 1913 (Ages 1621)

In his time within Hong Kong Ip forged a connection in Hong Kong with Leung Bik. Leung Bik was a child of Grandmaster Leung Jan. He had been studying with him for 4 years until his untimely loss of life.

1914 1937 (Ages 21 44)

The year 1914 was the time when Lp sought out the help of his brother LP Gai Gak to continue his studies at Kobe, Japan. With the support of his brother, the move was not a success. He ended up in the army and then became police officer. Ip Man was married to a woman with the name Cheung Wing Sing and together they had two daughters and two sons. The names were Ip Hok Ching, Ip Hok Chun, Ip Ar Sum, and Ip Ar Woon.

In his free time when he was not working, he would get together with his fellow martial artists and study each other's Kung Fu skills. For the sake of their education, according to reports, the instructor even put up an actual wooden dummy in the living space. The comrades that studied with him were Ip Chung Hong Yuan Kay Shan, Yiu Choi Tong-Gai as well as Lai Hip Chi. It was partly due to his dedication that Ip Man began to develop his own fan base throughout South China during the same time.

1937 (Age 44) The year 1937 (age 44) that the Japanese invading China which changed the lives of a lot of marital artists such as Ip Man.

1937 1945 (Ages 44 52)

In the time of this war, Ip Man struggled to stay within Foshan and live a simple daily. In spite of his career choice, Ip was determined to never allow his country's Japanese government to exploit his talents for causes that he did not agree. This meant that he could quickly find himself in financial disaster. His close friend Chow Chuen, was able to provide assistance when necessary. In order to repay the debt, he would instruct Kung Fu to Chow Kong Yiu's son.

1941 1943 (Ages 48 50)

Despite financial hardships however, he was capable of spending on spending more time to pursue his love of martial art. The time he spent in Luen Cheung's Luen Cheung Cotton Mill on Wing On Road as a teacher of Wing-Chun Kuen and other martial arts to a variety of enthusiastic students. One of the first was Ng Ying, Kwok Fu, Chow Kong Yiu, Chan Chi Sun, Lun Kai as well as Chow Sai.

1945 (Age 52)

Ip Man as well as the remainder of China will now breathe huge sighs of relief after Japan has surrendered, thus and brings the war in Asia to an end.

1945 1949 (Ages 54 56)

In the last few months, he has been more active than before. Because of time limitations, he had to stop his Wing-Chun class in addition to coaching Pang Nam as part of the Shung-Sha-Cheung-Yee Athletic-Association. Despite his busy schedule, his relationships with Tong-Gai as well as Pang-Nam meant that it was impossible to keep this obligation.

1950 1953 (Ages 57 60)

After a visit from Hong Kong in July of 1950, Ip Man makes a contact through Lee Man to obtain a teaching position in Tai Lam Street in Shamshuipo, Kowloon. The first class he taught at the new facility was shown at his Restaurant Workers Association. Leung Sheung as well as Lok Yiu attended the intimate training. The future students of his will comprise Ip Bo Ching Lee See Wing, Tsui Sheung Tin, and Man Siu Hung, Chiu Wan, and Law Ping. In the future, Ip Man would be transported to the headquarter of the Restaurant Workers Union in Sheung Wan in Hong Kong Island. Some of the notable people who took part in his training there included Yue Mei King Lee Wing, and Lee Ngan Foon.

1953 1954 (Ages 60 61)

Ip Man's class is moved from Tan Street. His pupils include Wong-Shun-Leung and Wong-Chok as well as Ng-Chan. The teacher taught private lessons to students. One of them was Lee Hon, at the 3 Princes Temple.

1954 1955 (Ages 61 62)

In this period, the school was actually relocated to its original location in The Restaurant Workers Union Headquarters in Sheung Wan. The most famous colleagues would be now included in Lo-Man Kam, Lee-Kam Sing, Cheung-Cheuk Hing and Kan-Wah Jeet (sometimes popularly referred to as the Victor Kan).

1955 1957 (Ages 6264)

Again, Ip Man's school changes site and it's this time it is now Lee-Tat St. in Yaumatei, Kowloon. Apart from the legend Lee-Siu-Lung (better called Bruce Lee) his pupils include Chan-Shin and Chow-Tze Chuen and Pang-KamFat. They also had Cheung-Hok Kin (Hawkin-Cheung) Siu-Yuk-Man and Poon-Ping Lid.

1957 1962 (Ages 64 69)

It is now located on Li Cheng Uk Estate. Li Cheng Uk Estate. In this stage, Ip Man is primarily offering private, one-on-one tuition in a range of locations. You can find him in

The Shun Kei pottery shop in Shaukeiwan training Wong-Bak Yee, Yeung-Chung Hon as well as Wong-Kwok-Yau. You can also see him at Po Lak Hong, Tsimshatsui teaching Tong-Cho-Chi in the form of Chan-Tak-Chi or Tam-Lai. In addition, he was present on TaiPo Rd. instructing Chung-Kam-Chuen and Chung-Wing-Hong.

1962 1963 (Ages 69 -70)

A different move has the school inside an Hing Ip Building at 61 Tai Po Road in Shamshuipo. Students attending classes could have been Chan Luen Lam, Cheung Yiu Wing, Chan Tai Yim, Ho Luen, Cheung Ching On, and Kwok See Yan. Additionally, Ip Man also led private instruction in Wah Tailor Shop. Wah Tailor Shop in Tsimshatsui.

1963 1965 (Ages 70 72)

Ip Man sees the school by way of a final move to the topmost floor in Tai Sang Restaurant which was situated at Fook Chuen Street in Taikoktsui. This particular area had previously been storage space. Ip's friend and close associate Ho Luen was kind enough to lend the room to continue education. Most of the pupils at the new facility included students from Ho Luen's Hing Ip Building. Alongside these students, Ip Man also found himself instructing other people, including police officers at an area on Hin Hing Street in San Po Kong.

1965-72 (Ages 72-79 years old)

The school was officially disbanded. Ip lived in the apartment he shared located on Tung Choi Street. With his increasing old age and was perhaps less agile than he was in earlier time, Ip had somewhat retired from his job as a teacher of Kung-Fu. There were still a lot of students who were still seeking his knowledge. So, he continued to train certain individuals most of them in his personal residence.

Also, Ip Man is believed for conducting training at three different places. When the Ving Tsun Athletic Association (the first government-registered martial arts society) first welcomed Wing-Chun classes, Ip Man stepped up to administer classes. At the time there was a team of instructors comprising Cheung-Ching-On, Fung Hon, and Wong-Hon would provide some of the instruction and instruction. On occasion, he would be instructing at Chan Kai Hong's house located on Waterloo Road . The most recent training offered through Ip Man was with Siu Fai Toi at Ip Sing Cheuk's residence.

1972 (Age 79)

In the month of December 1972 Ip Man passed away in his house in Tong Choi Street. Today, his last home in Fanling is sought-after from Martial Art enthusiasts.

Chapter 4: Yin And Yang

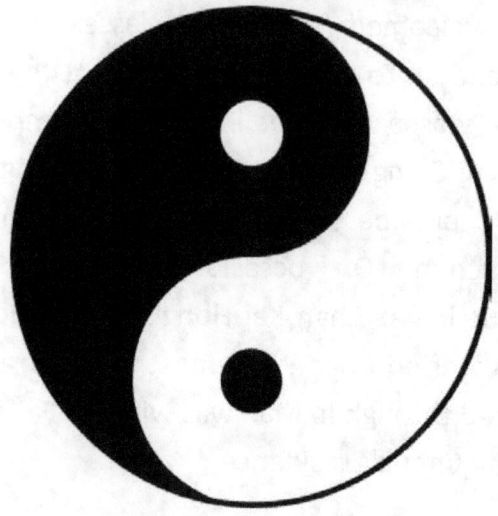

The concept that there is Yin and Yang is an essential philosophy for China as a whole, however it is also a specific application as well as numerous references to Martial Arts, even those that aren't from China that may not be referring to it in this way but agree with the underlying idea.

It is essentially Yin and Yang is used to define the dual nature of the universe that is, how opposing forces or opposite forces are present while being interconnected and dependent on one the other. This principle is so strong that it suggests that opposing forces linked, but they, in some instances, also give birth to one another.

One of the most obvious examples is one of day and night. The one cannot exist without others and they each give an opportunity to the other. Similar instances include cold and hot darkness and light, existence and death. (Most instances are natural).

For the martial Artist this concept is evident through the simplest Kung Fu salute or bow. The hand that is open and the closed fist is a further demonstration of Yin and Yang, masculine and feminine.

However, it can also be applied for training techniques. It is crucial to practice balance particularly in styles such as Kung Fu and Tai Chi which have the highest results achieved through a blend of both soft and hard techniques. both slow and quick.

This is an essential idea to consider when dealing with the opponent. If the attacker is threatening and uses a large amount of force, it is unwise to confront them using the same amount of force. Instead, the highly experienced martial Artist turns passive and applies the force of an attacker against them by using soft redirection to counter the hard force.

In a self-defense situation, you can counter an aggressive attacking high with a slick low kick, or the reverse.

Yin and Yang might seem as if they are esoteric concepts, however Martial Artists use it more often than it appears apparent.

Useful Terms in Wing Chun

This is a comprehensive list of distinctive terms one can come across in the practice of Wing-Chun. Each word is described in Chinese and is accompanied by as close to a exact translation as it is. Remember that the direct translation to English is only approximate, and pronunciations can vary.

Significant Terms and Techniques

Ng-Mui, a Buddhist born in the Siu Lim Temple. Her name is regarded as the founder of Wing-Chun.

(Ip) (Ip) Yip Man: An ardent teacher of the style that has been dubbed the "grandmaster" of Wing-Chun. His contribution was crucial for spreading this style and which in turn helped to ensure its continued development.

Basic Terms

Bart-Cham-Dao: Eight Slashing Butterfly Knives

Biu-Tze (Third Form): Finger Thrusting Form

Bok: Shoulder

Chuie: Punch or Blow

Chum-Kuu (Second Form): Arm or Bridge Seeking Form

Da: Strike

Dai: Lower Level of Defense or Attack

Dao: Knife

Jarn: Elbow Area

Jung: Palm Area

Jung-Sin: Your center line is the place that your actions are directed toward an opponent, and the location that you keep the best equilibrium and control of the body of yours

Kuen: Fist

Luk-Dim-Boon-Kwun: Six and One-half Point Pole, or Dragon-Pole Form

Ma: Stance

Muk-Yan-Chong is a form that uses an dummy made of wood.

Noi-Moon: The outer gate, or in the region between your arms

Oi-Moon is the outer gate or area between the outer and inner shoulder

Sau: Hand, or Arm

Sifu: Teacher, Master, or Guardian

Siu-Lim-Tao (First Form): Small Idea Form

Sut: Knee

Blocks and Deflections

Bong Sau: Wing Arm (Use the pinkie the wrist's side.)

Bie-Gee: Propelling the fingers and hands (Use the pinkie side on your wrist.)

Dai-Bong Sau: Low Wing Arm (Use the pinky finger side of your wrist.)

The Fak-Sau is a Whipping the Hand and Arm (Use by putting your finger on the pinkie the wrist.)

Fan-Sau Returning Hand (Bring your hands inwards to an enguarding place.)

Fook-Sau: Repressing the hand and arm (Use by placing your forearm on your thumb.)

Fut-Sau: Swinging Hands and Fingers (Use with the pinkie fingers part of your arm.)

Get-Sau A Slicing Hand or Sickle (Pull your hands in order to hold your bridge.)

Gum-Sau: Pinning Hand (Block by putting your elbow to the side of your own body.)

Huen-Sau: Revolving hand as well as arm (Use the wrist.)

Jip-Sau: Arm Break (Use Jut Sau and Tok Sau to "control the bridge".)

Jum-Sau What is a Sinking Hand? (Use the pinky finger the forearm's side)

Jut-Sau: Jerking hand or Arm (Strike with close-range power.)

Kau-Sau: Sickle hand (Control your adversaries bridge using your fingers.) Kwan Sau the Circling hands (Free yourself from the tension by turning you arms.)

the Lan-Sau Obstruction Arm or Bar Arm (Forearm and sometimes the palm)

The Lap-Sau is a method of controlling arm, or Seizing Arm (Used to grip more control of the hand.)

Mun-Sau: Hand of Questioning (Use your hands to protect the body's front.)

Man-Geng Sau: Neck-Pull hand (Refer to the discussion on Dummies.)

PakSau: Slap-Hand (Gather the power of your opponent by slapping them with the palm of the hand.)

Tan-Sau Tan-Sau (Make contact with your hand's thumb.)

Tok-Sau: The Rising Palm (Raise an unclosed palm and block.)

The Tuet-Sau method freeing hand (Hand posture derived from final of Siu Lim Tao.)

Wu-Sau: Hand Guard (Your hands is held that you can shield your body from an attack on the rear.)

Chi-Sau

Chi-Sau: Double Sticky Hands

Chi-Gerk: Sticky Legs

Dan-Chi-Sau: Single Sticky Hand

Poon-Sau: Rolling style Sticky Hands (natural movement)

Luk-Sau: Rolling style Sticky Hands (forward movement)

Gor-Sau: Free-Hand Movements

Closed-Fist Strikes

Chuen-Chuie: Inch Punch (A short-range Internal style punch)

Chung-Chuie: Thump-Punch (A powerful strike that is made with the hand that is posterior)

Fung-AnChuie: Phoenix Eye Punch (A strike in which the index finger is bent)

Jik-Chung-Chuie Straight (simple) punch (Fundamental linear strike)

"Lin-Wan-Kuen Chain-Punches (A combination of punches performed with a continuous stream)

Chapter 5: Open Palm Strikes

Dai-Jeung: A gentle strike with the palm that of your hand.

Chan-Jeung is a technique of hitting the head of an opponent or their upper torso using the edges of your hand, with the palm pointing upwards.

Jing-Jeung: a strike using the palm facing forward and up.

Pau-Jeung: A striking with your palm directed downwards and straight.

Wang-Jeung : This strike utilizes the sides of your palm to strike the upper or head of your opponent while keeping the hand facing downwards.

Elbow Strikes

GwaiJarn: The elbow is directed diagonally and pointed towards the ground.

Kup-Jarn In this exercise, your elbow points towards the ground, while you twist the remainder part of your body.

Pai-Jarn: The arm is pointed horizontally, and pointing towards your body.

Kicks

Chai-Gerk: Crescent or Stepping Kick

Chou-Gerk: Snapping Front Kick

Wang-Gerk: Side Kick or Horizontal Kick

Footwork

Biu-Ma: Thrusting Footsteps

Huen-Ma: Circling Footstep

Sam-Gwok-Ma: Three-Sided Triangle Footstep

Traditional Sequences

Inner/Outer Gate

Biu-Da: This technique involves a thrusting arm in combination with the striking hand

Guan-Da: A low and broad-swept block is joined by an attack with the opposing hand.

Tan-Da: One of the hands allows one hand to strike with the other hand while holding blocks with their palms directed upwards.

Outer Gate

Gum-Da: One hand hits the other and the other holds them down.

Huen-Da: A strike is made while the other arm is able to initiate a rotation in order to form large circles.

Lap-Da: One arm manages the opponent, and another hand prepares to strike.

Pak-Da: In this pattern, a strike is achieved by an arm block and an upward motion.

Miscellaneous Vocabulary

Bong: Wing

Biu: Thrusting Motion

Dantien: Ones energy center. The Dantien can be located about two inches over the navel, also known as the belly button.

Fa-Ging: Release Power

Fak: Quick Sweeping Movement

Fan: Return

Fook: Gain Control

Fut: Fling About

Gee: Fingers

Gong-Lik: The Energy Source From Within

Gum: Pinning or Pressing

-Guan to split, break or break into pieces of two or more.

Huen: Rotate Around

Jip: Single Jerking/Lifting Motion

Jum: Fall or Lower

Jut: Jerking Movement

Kau: Short and Swinging Strike

Lan: Block the movements of an opponent.

Lap: Gain Control

Man: Questioning

Pak: Evade a Blow

Sau: Arm

Tan: Widening -

Tok: Lifting or Raising

Tues: Exemption from Restrictions

Yee-Chi-Kim-Yeung-Ma: Core Position for Wing-Chung

Ying and Yang: Complimentary Opposites. Male and Female, Logic and Creativity, or Active and Passive

Wu: Protect

Wing-Chun Blocks and Applications

Blocks

Below, you'll find an explanation of every block of Wing-Chung. They are supported by an general English translation. It also discusses their weaknesses and strengths as well as suggested uses. Each block is named after the way in the other blocks. As a matter of fact they can be thought of as deflections. This feature can be traced to Wing-Chun's indirect block theory. It is essential to bear this at the forefront when learning about the methods in this section.

Though each block is beneficial, they are only useful when they are used within the proper contexts. It's not feasible for a single position or move to provide complete security. But, if you combine both the highs and lowers, and the inner and outer are likely to build a very effective system of protection.

Bong Sau (Winged Arm)

The very first method of blocking that we'll discuss is Bong Sau. It is a technique used to avoid direct strikes because the force of the striking force reaches the wrist. Students are taught to lower the Bong and thus create an opportunity for them to get closer to their attacker. If the punch is aimed closer to the elbow, the athlete is expected to be able adapt and lower the elbow to the Tan Sau.

It is crucial to maintain an eloquent posture when performing Bong Sau as a response to a straight strike raised. If you don't, you'll be unable to defeat your opponent and create an enormous advantage for the opponent. The body's relaxed position allows it to take on a higher strength than if your body is rigidly.

If you are attempting to stop a less straight strike, it's important to take the opposite form of shape. In this case, a rigid structure such as Dai Bong Sau, is better. If you were to loosen up your posture, your block would be uneffective and could be dangerous for your capacity to maintain stability. With a firm stance, you can effortlessly block your opponent's strike.

Bong Sau lets the user to move quickly between a striking and blocking place while retaining the elbow of your opponent. Bong Sau can be useful both in the outer and inner gates to be used interchangeably.

Application The Bong Sau deflection is appropriate to stay clear of high and low-impact punches. The primary benefit for this particular style is its ability to effortlessly transition into the next stance easily. It is also helpful in getting a feel for your opponent to gauge the strength of their intentions and determination. Its drawback is that it often leaves the shoulder susceptible to attacks. Additionally, it is not able to benefit of being able to defend and attack simultaneously.

Biu Sau (Thrusted Hand)

Biu Sau is the go option for staying clear of the direct impact on your skull or face. In this manner, you can effortlessly transition between the outer and inner gate, and then back to the inner one with a range of coordinated forms. When standing on the floor in Bui Sau your elbow needs to be pointed at your body. So, you're able to display a sense with power that can be a challenge to the opponent as well as your own centre.

Application: This advanced block can easily be adapted to the build of your opponent and the direction of the attack. Furthermore, Biu Sau can take the form of an offensive strike and can be executed by initiating the attacker with a sharp poke in the eyes of your attacker. It is important to note that one must only try Biu Sau after a sufficient amount of training. It's very easy to fall into yourself especially when it is paired by a skilled adversary. Also, it is ineffective when matched against blows that are less powerful.

Fak Sau (Whisking Hand)

The block that is loosely named "Whisking Hand" is utilized when two participants are within proximity to one another. It can be helpful if striking is made towards your neck or throat. It is actually not a deflection in the slightest but more an attack counter-attack. If your intention to attack your opponent is blocked, Fak Sau is an effective method to fool the enemy. When executed properly the move can have huge effect. Apart from being an efficient way of avoiding the impact of a punch, this move can be employed to carry out the direction change without falling off the balance.

Application Application: The Fak Sau technique is used to escape a battle in a restricted zone. It is a method to maintain the space of a large area while shifting directions. The movement demands a lot of attention as well as the ability to anticipate approaching attacks from multiple perspectives.

Fook Sau (Suppressing Hand)

Fook Sau defense is unique in that it does not have a specific purpose. Fook Sau defense is unique because it is not built. It's not designed to defend against a specific kind of attack. It is more of an intermediary to move across a stance. The flexibility of it makes it suitable for novices, but still beneficial to masters. This is a way of maintaining a relationship to your opponent and gaining control through anticipating the next action. Fook Sau can be distinguished from Fook Sau in other positions through repositioning your arm, by circling your hands.

Application: Because Fook Sau is really more of a strategy that allows you hand to be free to strike your own attacks against your adversary. It allows you to switch stances while not falling prey to being surprised. It's among the primary blocking techniques to be used by Wing-Chun students need to master.

Fut Sau (Flicking Hand)

As with Fook Sau, this technique is frequently used as an approach to get between positions. It is distinct in the fact that Fut Sau is performed with an opposite hand. The name derives due to the performer's skill in "flicking" around to evade any opponent's attack or stop the block, opening the ability to see their eyes are always vulnerable. It causes pain to opponents, which results in the opponent enough of a distraction that they can discover your opening and strike with a firm strike. It is crucial to assess how the enemy attempts to come at you. If they do so with sufficient strength, then chances of their move being unsuccessful are diminished. This technique is best used when you are in the outside gate. It is vital to be aware of getting that knowledge to be able to recognize the best time to adjust your strategies.

Applications: Fut Sau is ideal for influencing your adversaries' guard however, it could be unsuccessful in the event that their tactics are tooagresiv.

Gum Sau (Pinning Hand)

The pin can be useful for limiting the range of motion of an opponent's arm leg. It is only successful when both players have a good distance since it is required for the other to be in contact with each other. Gum Sau could be compared to a different Wing-Chun pin, which is known in the form of Lan Sau. It is a common practice using Gum Sau as a prelude that allows quick movements through Lan Sau to hold an arm in such a way that the person will have no chance to strike a punch or block.

Furthermore, Gum Sau works well when paired with a push driven by a shoulder. If someone else tries to grab the grip of your wrist it is possible that Gum Sau could be used as a team by a shoulder shove in order to disengage from the person who is attacking you. Additionally, this can provide an occasion to unleash the attack of your own. This kind of maneuver is best when performed starting from the outside gate.

Application: Apply Gum Sau to immobilize your adversaries' limbs. It's only effective if you're within distance. It is only able to block punches or stop an attack or kick. it is able to stop the kick.

Chapter 6: Splitting Hand

Guan Sau is another effective pin to defend against attacks. Similar to Gum Sau it is most efficient in close proximity. Also, it can be considered close relatives of the pin known as Lan Sau. Gum Sau is an effortless way to transition towards Lan Sau. This technique is great to block both high and low blows. It is also useful for avoiding the use of kicks. Incorporating an attack of your own is an excellent technique to combine defense with offensive. Guan Sau operates in both the gates of the outside and inside dependent on the type of movement it's coupled with. It is for instance, if you pair two distinct Guan Sau actions or just one Guan Sau using a lowered elbow, which is performed with Jum Sau. The masters of Wing-Chun can use Guan Sau to aid in the process of bending their adversaries and making them easier opponents.

Use: This pin can be extremely effective when used in conjunction with strike. It protects yourself from high and low strikes and stop kicks. However, it doesn't provide an adequate defense against a kick which is already moving.

Huen Sau (Turning Hand)

It is possible to maintain subtle contact against your opponent using the Huen Sau method. It can be helpful when you transition from one entrance into the next. This means that you'll be able to discern their intents and prepared to respond quickly. How it's done responds to the sensations in the wrist. Huen Sau can be described as a turn or circling motion that turns the gate.

Application: This technique works perfectly with a variety of forms, that make it useful to use in a variety of techniques. The speed with which Huen Sau is executed is a drawback since the performer has to compromise the strength. Huen Sau is not as effective when it comes to masters since they can easily recognize and overcome the move.

Jum Sau (Sinking Hand)

Jum Sau is akin to the Tan Sau method, except it's performed with the opposite arm. It is accomplished through blocking the direction of the striker's arm using your own and directing it away from the direction it was intended to go. Because the posture used similar to many Wing-Chun strikes, it is possible to switch from a block strikes effortlessly. In addition, martial artists may shift from Jum Sau to the Lan Sau pin with just some simple adjustments. The versatile block works within both the inner and out gate and is able to be easily switched between the two.

Application: The process of executing Jum Sau is similar to a normal punch. However, you don't hit your person you are fighting. It allows you to shift through a range of positions swiftly.

Jut Sau (Jerking Hand)

The majority of martial arts systems employ an exact technique for speeding the body's muscles, thereby creating more strength. For instance, in Karate the students learn to slightly twist their wrists as they execute a punch. Wing-Chun's method to this problem is Jut Sau. Jut Sau is particularly effective for close-quarters work. It is able to join any type of motion that includes strikes. It should never be employed in punching as should you make a mistake, then there's a high chance of causing injury to the wrist. For those who have Wing-Chun masters skilled enough to perform the task proficiently, this punch is extremely efficient.

Another method to use Jut Sau is by striking the opponent's hand or arm to force them to get out of the way. Jut Sau is effective in both the gates that are both outer and inside.

Applications: Jut Sau is considered to be a highly advanced shorter-range strike. Also, it is a technique to increase the impact. Though extremely effective, Jut Sau requires ample time and commitment to master, which is why it's classified as a technique for Wing-Chun that is considered to be advanced.

Kwan Sau (Rotating Arm)

The skill can be practiced using it using the Dummy and Bie-Gee positions. Kwan Sau is an advanced skill, making it ideal for those who have extensive training in Wing-Chun. If Kwan Sau is performed in the motion, each hand is intended to turn in such an order that they will eventually swap gates. This will give yourself the chance to hit your opponent.

A majority of instructors combine this method with an additional Guan Sau. It is possible to follow with any of a variety of positions typically accompanied by an Jum Sau when in the event of high attacks or Low Gran Sau to attempt a low strike.

The circular motions allow for many more actions, and prevents the opponents from doing their own as well as aids in keeping or maintaining balance on in the middle line. The legend says Kwan Sau employs two hands in order to make one perfect strike.

Lan Sau (Obstruction Arm)

Lan Sau is the most important instrument to create more distance between the practitioner and their adversary. The range at which this technique can be most effective is also the minimal area needed for Wing-Chun's hand position and strike. If the players are in very close proximity, then Lan Sau could be utilized in order to get back control.

Lan Sau is a good all-around partner of Bong Sau, which acts as an easy transition into this method. If used in conjunction, one is in a position to pull their attacker's arms around their body and then have the chance to hit them.

In some cases, Lan Sau is also translated into "Arm Bar". In lieu of grappling with the opponent, this technique can be used to keep an appropriate distance to get a wider flexibility of motion. This is usually done in conjunction with diverse hand strategies. The outer gate Lan Sau works well at pining an opponent's arms. However, it could be employed in the inner gate to hold an opponent's throat.

The application: Lan Sau is a method of creating an area larger for work. It also shows the minimum space required for Wing-Chun. Additionally, Lan Sau is an effective pin but isn't an effective blocking technique. It is important to be careful not to transfer between Lan Sau to an intense wrestling situation.

Lap Sau (Deflecting Arm)

When an alternate hand strategy uses to make contact to the opponent, the technique of Lap Sau can be considered a vital ability. The technique is performed by fast, but powerful pull on the arm. It forces them to move away from the center of their body for a brief moment, providing the chance to hit.

Lap Sau is a great way to increase the force of a strike, especially when you are in close proximity. The potential of deflecting and striking at the same time is referred to as "two-way power". The technique works only at the gate's outermost. It's risky to try Lap Sau within the inner gate because it's hard to control the direction the opponent's movements are influenced, thereby increasing chances of them colliding onto you or affecting your position.

Application Lap Sau: Lap Sau technique is achieved through pulling an opponent's arms and forcing them to lose balance. While technically, it's not an attack, it can be extremely effective at getting an advantage over the opponent. It is however challenging to master against an opponent that is substantially larger than your opponent since this will require greater force and poses a threat of injury to your core.

Mun Sau (Asking Hand)

Mun Sau is the leader of Wu Sau in the Wing-Chun guard. The purpose of this guard is to make contact to your opponent as you transition to a different posture. By holding your hands in Mun Sau will stop your opponent from having the ability to read the intentions of your hand. It could be distracting from the attack. Mun Sau is a form of martial arts where Mun Sau the hand is put directly in front of your body. This leaves less space for you to cover to make a strike that is successful.

Useful: Mun Sau is your primary defense. It blurs your opponent's vision, allowing for an instant reflex. Masterful Wing-Chun practitioners can employ Mun Sau to nudge their opponents out in the light. However, any advantage comes risk, the most obvious in this instance, the chance that your opponent will grab or pining your arms.

Pak Sau (Slapping Arm)

Pak Sau can be a strategy to conceal your motives which is usually utilized in conjunction with Fak Sau. Its primary goal is to defend against attacks. It also has the possibility of creating greater distance between you with your opponent. Pak Sau easily transitions to Gum Sau that pins your attacker's arms. Even with these benefits, it's crucial to keep in mind that Pak Sau isn't usually suited to blockincoming strikes. If you do, the chance of a miscalculated timing, not making the strike and later having your limb damaged is just too risky.

However, it does well against attempts to grab or close grappling. It is therefore efficient in both the gates that are both outer and inside. Pak Sau is usually thought of as being a way to transform to other forms, as it is in the case of Gor Sau and Chi-Sau.

Application: This method can be used to gain access to the attacker through opening up space, stopping captures and clouding their vision. Also, it is a great tool to transition for other forms of combat as well as being a method that can be executed swiftly. This isn't the ideal form for preventing strikes.

Tan Sau (Open-Hand)

Tan Sau is one of the primary techniques employed in Wing-Chun, which in reality connects Bong Sau as well as Fook Sau to form "the Three Seeds". If you are targeted in a way that is close to the elbow, Tan Sau can be utilized to defend. The technique can be very effective for defending the front portion of your body. If an opponent is able to connect with your body through the Tan Sau posture it is easy to move your elbow towards Bong Sau in order to block any attempt.

Tan Sau can also allow the use of a hand that is free for you to inflict pain on your adversary. The real benefit from this strategy is the ability to protect and annoy simultaneously. When combined, both the Tan Sau arm as well as the free arm are able to protect the line of center while keeping both elbows towards the ground.

In the gate's outer area in the outer gate, the arm acting is raised above the elbow of the opponent. If working inside the gate, that arm must be placed below the elbow of the opponent. The result is that they will be not able to bend their arms to strike properly.

Applications: Tan Sau can be utilized to take control of the attacker. Its strength is due to its capability to stop and start an attack while at the same time. If you are close to your wrist, Tan Sau's its effectiveness.

Tok Sau (Elbow Lifting Hand)

According to its name, this strategy is based on raising the elbow. Tok Sau can be used to raise an opponent's arm close to their elbow. There is a good chance that Wing-Chun depends on building strength over the opponent. One of the most efficient strategies to accomplish this is to limit the movement of the arms. This is because the elbows are the primary reason for this type of control. Tok Sau can be used in situations where an adversary is pushing your arm and you must regain control before they can push the other person over.

Do Tok Sau, by lifting your opposing arm and elbow. It alters the direction of their force to flow upwards and down on your body. This causes you to are heavier and more solid.

Another method to utilize Tok Sau could be to use it to break your opponent's weight. The same manner, with the opponent lifting their elbows up. The move helps to reduce their shape. Both times, Tok Sau only operated within the gate's outer perimeter.

Application: Through pushing or pulling onto the elbow of an opponent Tok Sau can help them gain balance and builds your. This technique is great when combined with Jut Sau where the objective is to break completely the elbow joint (Jip Sau). This technique isn't an attempt to deflect, nor can it be employed to stop the threat of a strike. It is merely a means to manipulate your opponents arms to your advantage.

Wu Sau (Guarding Hand)

Wu Sau makes up an important component of the Wing Chun guard. This technique requires that the guarding hand is positioned in the direction of the leading hand which is Man Sau. If the dominant hand gets taken away or seized by a tyrant, the Wu Sau guard hand will be used as a backup option of defense.

Applications: Wu Sau offers additional protection against the opponent. This is not so effective against a skilled Wu-Chun player as they could use this method to advantage. Make sure they do not try to force you into a Chi Sau or Gor Sau posture that they are able to master.

The Wing Chun Forms

Many martial art styles employ the patterns, forms or "Katas to some extent or the other. In Wing-Chun they are the elements used to master every move or method. In contrast to other martial arts that may require hours of intense learning, Wing-Chun only has a handful of forms that you can remember.

A simpler system, with less forms to learn and allows students to devote greater time to practice each move until the movement becomes instinctual. There is no need to memorize difficult sequences like it is in other martial art. The core of Wing-Chun is three of the open hand styles.

Siu Lim Tao

Chum-Kiu

Biu Tze (Bie Gee)

When the open hand poses after mastering them the student of Wing-Chun can begin to learn how to perform the exercises using the wooden dummy. Also, they will be taught the two weapons forms referred to in the form of Pole or Butterfly Sword. Each tool or form allows to perform a variety of tasks with different positions. Students must be aware of the right positioning and usage for each type of form. When they have learned, a student may return to basic forms and learn how every new instrument or method is used.

My personal experience with various forms of martial arts have proven that all forms are capable of a wide range of interpretations, Wing-Chun is no exception. Every single student as well as Martial Arts master develops their unique method for utilizing traditional methods. There is a possibility of differences in the best method of application. The perception one has of each type and their best application can change with time. The greater clarity in the purpose can be found only after committed training. The more time one spends studying Wing-Chun and the more one can comprehend.

The people who learn Wing-Chun have the exact same style of practice. They can be found in different forms and sizes. They are not all born from the same conditions or brought to the martial arts similar ways. It's therefore expected that the method by how we apply every tool is similarly varied. This is one of the reasons of the necessity for different forms to be taught in different stages of the process of learning, in order to build upon a range of theories that are converging.

As with everything else in life The complexity of Wing-Chun is enhanced with each new lesson. The same is true for the level of one's knowledge. Siu Lim Tao is a element used to aid students in their beginning stages learn fundamental actions. Later, more complicated types like Biu Tze or the Muk Yan Chong (Wooden Dummy) can be used to help teach more complicated methods. If the more complex techniques were introduced to an untrained student, they could only confuse and frustrate them without any benefit. It is best to teach them only once the student is ready to master them.

In order to master each Wing-Chun practice, the student is required to go into the state of mind that is different. Like meditation, the mind becomes free of any distracting thoughts. It is essential to have a clear and focused mind to be able to concentrate on the specifics of any activity.

Though it may appear simple on surface, every form really a result of a thought that may include 100 different movements all at once. The good news is that many of these actions can be described as the result of repeated actions. Through repetition that you can achieve perfection. This is especially beneficial in attempting to master most complex methods. The ability to practice is what can transform one's initial uncoordinated movements into a perfect technique.

Keep in mind at the core of the Wing-Chun philosophy lies the simplicity. To make every lesson clear each shape is broken down into its most basic form. Each one is mastered at an time followed by a re-union into a beautifully arranged performance.

An Overview of Siu Lim Tau

Wing-Chun's first and most earliest structure was titled Sui Lim Tau which essentially is "Little idea". As with Siu Lim Tau, small ideas are able to be transformed to larger, more complex entities that serve a the greatest significance. Actually, this description could encompass as much as 90% of the hand-based techniques of Wing-Chun.

Instructors employ Siu Lim Tau as a tool to instruct their students beyond hand-skills. Siu Lim Tau is also utilized to teach beginners about concepts of balance and energy which includes the central line. This class teaches you to use the inner as well as the outer gates.

Siu Lim Tau requires a static positioning. There's no movement or feetwork required. Instead, focus is to stand in a steady position, keeping a specific pattern. It is important to find how to anchor yourself on the floor beneath. This way, the participant can gain more force and control from the hips.

In the end, the structure can be used to teach students in four directions. They include the front back and two sides. It is important to be aware of the different zones and know how to defend each one while provoking the attack of your own.

One of the main themes in Wing-Chun is the capacity to increase your power over the opponent through positioning your elbow in a certain way. These adjustments will also ensure your center line gets stronger.

Chapter 7: The Basics Of Siu Lim Tau

Lesson One

The initial Siu Lim Tau lesson for the student to master will be the starting posture. It is the basis of the entire posture. The stance is set so that knees are bent a bit and toes on the feet are dispersed to ensure the balance. The position mimics the shape of an arc. Based on the laws of physics, it evenly distributes your load of your body onto every foot.

It is essential to devote sufficient time on this lesson in order to fully grasp every aspect. This will be extremely helpful to students when they are able to learn the new methods later. Concentrate on every structure and the connection between the elbow and forearm. All power must originate from your elbow, and not from the entire arm.

It is also the time that instructors help each student identify and increase the power of their arms and wrists. While performing the exercise, most of the effort will come at the elbow. The muscles of the triceps will have to stay taut during any motion that pushes like the one employed for Fook as well as Tan Sau. Similar to this the bicep muscles must remain flexed while the arm are being pulled back as when Wu Sau is being used.

The connection between your feet and the hips is vital. When you push, for example the movements in Tan Sau or Fook Sau the hips have to be leaning towards the front, and the weight of your body is transferred towards the ball of the feet. In contrast, maintaining your balance by pulling, such as Wu Sau demands the hips to be pressed to the back and weight is shifted to the heels. Learning these techniques can help novices stay grounded and be able to withstand the force or pulling of the adversary. With the help of adjusting your hips, and feet, they will also discover how to redirect the adversaries' energies.

The initial lesson concludes by introducing Pak Sau. The position is at an angle of 45 degrees away from the middle line of your body. This can be accomplished by using the upright palm strike. Be aware of the position of your elbow, which has focus to one side away from your body. This prevents the opponent's limb from crushing or hitting the opponent. Pak Sau can be employed to strike an opponent through the gate inside.

Lesson Two

The next part should be taught in a slow and deliberate speed. Every step must be completed smoothly and in a precise method. Both the teacher and student are likely to spend the majority of their time looking at the postures as well as the power they require. The techniques taught during the second session need practice both ways and not just because they're dual handed, but rather to develop the strength to do these exercises using whichever arm is at ease.

They work in both the outer and the inner gates. The instructor will teach you the ability to quickly change from one position to the following. It is achievable due to the manner in which each hand move can be linked to the next.

Alongside understanding the postures the lesson can also assist the student to build power, control as well as speed. The ones who achieve the greatest performance will be those that are able to keep an equilibrium throughout. This will reduce the amount of force which can make each step slower.

Lesson Three

This lesson from Siu Lim Tau focuses on maintaining the center line as well as producing forward-moving energy. The lesson begins with Pak Sau, which is accompanied by the open hand strike, which is positioned at a 45-degree angle away from the body. The elbow stays pointed towards the ground. Utilize this posture to defend any attack coming from the outside gate. Because of the elbow's angle, it allows the practitioner to grip the attacker's arms, giving them an opportunities to strike.

Then, there is the hand position. Every one of them is performed with a certain distance from the ground. Learning the proper hand postures will allow the students to defend against attacks at any angle. The way to defend is similar however being able to change your position in relation to the opponent is one of the most important skills.

The student then is able to recognize how to move between gates. For practice teachers will introduce the student to Bong Sau Tan Sau. If the entire Siu Lim Tau can be merged, it is possible to fight from a myriad of strikes using a single hand by shifting from one position and back again, with a focus upon the arm.

The student then is taught how to dislodging an opponent when he is able to hold their wrist. For a beginner, this move could appear like a strike. The technique works by striking the attacker's hand while liberating your hand. But, according to Wing-Chun theorem, it's much more efficient to attack your adversary with your free hand instead of wasting energy trying to release the opponent.

An Overview of Chum-Kiu

The second version of Wing-Chun is known as Chum-Kiu. The English translation of the Chinese word results in "arm searching shape" as well as "seeking for the bridge". In this class, one can learn more complex techniques, forms, as well as energy methods. The Wing-Chun class is taught in a sequence with increasing difficulties. This means that the following lesson will always be a little higher in difficulty than the previous. The case with Chum-Kiu this can be explained by the inclusion of footwork in the forms. One concept that is based on the proper use of feet, is that of distance.

In this part, the kicks are joined by hand movements, resulting in an improved technique of Wing-Chun. All of these must cooperate for a more balanced balance of body weight. They should not exceed the waist of a player. This would cause energy and power loss.

The Basics of Chum-Kiu

Lesson One

The first lesson of Chum-Kiu is focused on the distribution of weight. To achieve an optimal balance of weight it is necessary for the learner to stand with their feet further apart as opposed to Siu Lim Tao. This ensures stability during rotation or twisting motions, and permits easier adjustments.

Once you have mastered the new posture and turning easily The next step is straightening the arms to a Fut Sau posture. The method is to apply stress on the elbows. Both arms are now able to unite, creating an end to the opponent's arm.

Then, the beginner in Wing-Chun gets introduced to moves with new direction. It is then mastered by practicing Lan Sau as well as Bong Sau. Apart from being a powerful attack tool, Lan Sau can also be employed as a defense tool. Combining these two forms allows the pupil to move closer to the opponent and then hold their arms.

The end of the lesson's first part is to understand the concept of energy in two ways. The ability to master this can provide additional energy to your work.

Lesson Two

In the next section, Chum-Kiu's pupil will be able to add the skill of stepping into their arsenal. The goal is to improve from the lessons previously taught that focus on the arm and foot. For beginners, the most difficult part in martial arts is to ensure that your whole body is in synch. In the event of a mishap, it can significantly weaken one's defense.

The practice of kicks is an effective method to keep the adversaries in check. In some cases, they are used for closing distances or making a move forward in order to meet the adversary. So the phrase, "seeking the bridge" is a perfect fit for the situation.

Bong Sau is particularly important at this time. When a wrist is trapped, the wrist can utilize your elbows. The practice is commonly referred to as "emergency Bong Sau". In the end, students will be taught on ways to increase their control on the line of center. It is best to practice shifting between Bong Sau as well as striking or Jum Sau posture.

Lesson Three

The Chum-Kiu final lesson starts with a particular type of kick. It is useful in cutting down distance between the instructor and their adversaries. Also, it can be used as an effective method to keep opponents away.

Then, follow with an lowered two Bong Sau. In order to complete the sequence, most instructors prefer an lowered Tan Sau. When performing the low Bong Sau the student stays in a tight position as a form to protect themselves. A relaxed posture at this point could render the body at risk. After that, the Tan Sau must be relaxed in order to permit the body to move more freely.

In the end, Chum-Kiu demonstrates the method of overcoming an attempt to hold your throat. The person must also make a backward step as they strike the hold. The method is the double Jut Sau. The double palmed blow is followed by wrists being twisted in a way that the backs the hands are facing to the other direction. The arms are twisted backwards in what is called the reading place.

After that, the person walks backward before turning so that they are also facing in towards the other direction. Making these turns will help the pupil to keep the proper balance of weight during every move. This Wu Sau technique taught in this section also shows how to block and turn simultaneously time.

An Overview of Bie-Gee (Biu Tze)

A Bie-Gee interpretation can lead one to a phrase that reads, "thrusting fingers". The part that refers to this in Wing-Chun can be utilized to explain a range of subjects. There are higher-level stances, moves as well as energy concepts. Also, it covers the manner that all these instruments can be combined to create an unbeatable attack against the opponent, thereby increasing their power and decreasing the effort they exert to attack.

Chapter 8: The Basics Of Bie-Gee

Lesson One

Bie-Gee has a unique method of tackling your adversary. This is known as Pie Jarn. The most simple description of it is in three terms, namely it is a "hacking elbow hit". Pie Jarn is used to perform turning motions. It is accomplished by lifting one hand up and quickly lower it until the elbow is in contact with the adversary. It is important to understand that the Pie Jarn movement requires intimate distance between you and your opponent.

Apart from having a practical instrument, Pie Jarn demonstrates how to remedy imbalance that is caused by a frenzied block or strike. Bong Sau is closely connected with Pie Jarn because creating the Biu Sau movement beneath Bong Sau could also restore control over that center line.

In the event that the two Biu Sau's are placed with one on top and the other underneath, you is likely to notice an obvious capability to move between gates. It is possible to commit what is commonly referred to as double Huen Sau, before returning both arms in the middle and rotating both legs, they can also resume the line of center.

In the beginning, Three Pie Jarn strikes must be used three times. The next lessons will demand to use them only once time. At first, there were three levels, so they were the first to use a repetition of three times, the next two, and the third was just one. But, Yip Man found it to not be necessary and therefore ended the middle tier.

Lesson Two

The Pie Jarn technique is now executed with the same sequence used in the previous lesson. It is different that the subsequent Biu Sau is replaced with an elevated palm strike. It is recommended to place the strike at an angle of 45 degrees relative towards the central line. Once you have mastered the technique, you can repeat the lesson, only this time by using a lower hand strike.

Lesson Three

The last Biu Sau lesson starts with Kum Sau. The sequence consists of Jum Sau as well as Guan Sau. A teacher should show how to do a rotational Kwun Sau. Start by moving to the left side and then to the right, and then return on the left side for a complete. It is a complicated move that includes both low and high strikes. Thus, the judo practitioner has the ability to keep the opponent guessing.

The idea is that in Kwun Sau each arm should be distinct and allow enough space to allow for motion. The final lesson of Biu Sau is used to show forms that change across the gates. An example of this is an oblong wooden model.

The student is also able to perform the three Fau Sau forms. They are distinct from the forms that were previously practiced within Siu Lim Tao or Chun Kiu. They raise to a forty-five degree angle. This small modification affects what is intended by Fau Sau, now it is a suitable advanced strike as well as offering protection from an attack from the sides.

While the traditional Fau Sau form is stationary however, some tweaks could give the guard's natural stance. This stance can also help align the line of center to swiftly come back from an attack. To find the correct position in a tense turn and rotate 90 degrees changing towards Fak Sau while dropping your elbow down just a bit.

Following a sequence of three Fak Sau's initial hand is expected to return to its centerline before it is lowered to Wu Sau. The hand then is moved out at the 45 degree angle in order to locate Fook Sau. For the final step, Huen Sau must be executed in order to return in a correct shape with a balanced posture as well as an unprotected center line.

This lesson is now geared towards another set of triples that this time that involves it in the Biu Sau form. When they bring their hands towards the center of their hand, the student pushes it in Biu Sau. While the second hand follows beneath the first hand, instigating the Biu Sau strike. This technique can be used as a method of an exercise to master how to master the Biu Sau structure and moving between two gates, while making sure to keep the central point.

In the 3rd grouping in this class is the Bie-Gee which is followed by the hand open for a strike. Similar to the first sequence we mentioned, this one incorporates a block as well as an attack. The sequence begins by raising a double Lap Sau that is then rotated to ninety degrees. The process is then followed by a palm strike or sometimes an upper-cut type punch.

At the end, the pupil will be introduced to an effective technique for relaxation, as successful execution of Bie Gee is heavily on this technique. In other words, it could become exhausting for beginners as it involves a variety of complicated movements. It is an instrument to regain one's composure after rapid reaction like being able to escape a blow or standing up after being thrown down.

Be aware that prior to rising to the top, both arms must form the form of a raised guard to safeguard the head as it will be the first area of your body to be lifted and should not be unprotected. The last lesson of Biu Sau will also concentrate on hip movements that are precise and will assist the student in breaking free from a gripping hold and gaining control over their adversaries.

An Overview of Chi-Sau (Sparring)

It is one of the most popular methods for gaining martial art proficiency. In Wing-Chun the practice which is done against an actual adversary is known as Chi-Sau, also known as "sticky-hands". The practice is based on basic arm postures like Bon-Sau-Tan-Sau-Tan-SauFook-Sau. In Chi-Sau the poses are executed with a roll-like way. The two participants control these movements by circling, moving both in the direction of forward and reverse.

The student is putting in practice the idea that the sensations of touch are more sensitive than vision. Students learn to trust their instinctual reacting to sensations without even seeing the situation. This is what gives Wing-Chun's famous speed. Through continuous Chi-Sau training, you can develop lightning-fast hand skills.

But, there is some limitations to this kind of expertise. You must have the ability to let go. An overly stressed body is reduced, therefore learning to achieve a state of relaxed is just as important as acquiring each technique.

Chi-Sau's aim is to train the student to fight in a real-world encounter. There is often an absence between learning an art of combat and the preparation to defend yourself from a potential threat. Chi-Sau can bridge that gap by allowing training with real opponents. It allows students to defend themselves fast and efficiently, if needed.

The importance of this practice is because of a prominent characteristic of Wing-Chun. Its reliance on the feeling of touch isn't one that we typically employ. It is a skill that must be mastered and refined through repeated use. The skill is not something that one is able to master in a single day, but it may take a lot of effort. Chi-Sau is an excellent method to master this skill.

Though Chi-Sau has been intended to simulate real-life situations, it doesn't include real punches or kicks. The focus on this type of training is to learn how to assess the opponents. It is the most effective method to master the ability to recognize energy levels and the instincts of your body, and to maintain equilibrium and stay in the middle line, in order to produce an explosive striking.

Although there are many theories about Wing-Chun, It is crucial to understand that the core of Wing-Chun is simplicity. The student should keep the concepts easy in their heads and a trained body can bring out the moves from memory. A sloppy display of bravado might be attractive to a crowd, however they're less effective than an easy, well-controlled defense.

The third force that is driving every form of Wing-Chun is the central line. If there is no stability that comes from following this line, opponents could quickly take full control during fighting. The process of navigating Chi-Sau can appear as an exchange. Students and teachers allow room to each other's ideas to develop. For analogy, there's the fine line between discussion or debate, and more fierce argument that should be not averted. If you try to dominate your opponent with Chi-Sau will defeat the main intention behind this technique.

As with "the three forms," there are different Chi-Sau levels arranged in the difficulty level. Students progress through these levels while becoming better at each activity.

Dan-Chi-Sau

Lok-sau/ Bong Lap Sau

Poon Sau

Luk Sau

Gor Sau

Dan-Chi-Sau (Single-Style Sticky Hands)

Dan-Chi-Sau is considered to be the very first and, therefore, most basic of Chi-Sau techniques. In this part where the student of Wing-Chun is exposed to a important aspect of this specific martial art system. Feeling can be a great resource for understanding how to strike, when to defend and how tough your opponent is.

Simple hand movements help focus the mind and focus on subtle changes in energy flow and. It is best to practice these together with a partner to show the mind and body how to cooperate and, as a result, they can mirror the movements of one another with ease.

The process of learning this technique will require a quantity of cooperation. Particularly, they'll try to determine where and the position of their arm situated without even looking. Each will attempt to predict the movement of their opponent in a way that matches them in direction, but also speed and force. A way of practicing Dan-Chi-Sau is by forming different positions using just one hand of each participant's.

Lok-Sau/Bong-Lap-Sau

The next level of Chi-Sau is the exercise known in the form of Lok-sau and Bong Lap Sau. As with the first exercise, this also utilizes Wing-Chun's simplest hand postures. But, the challenge increases with the addition of the footwork. In pairs, the students perform the strike. The second student places the hand into Bong Sau while rotating their feet. This rotation prepares them for the more strenuous footwork that is to come. The next student will use Lap Sau to stop the initial student's strike. Then they use their Bong Sau hands attempt to strike on the opposing center line. At the conclusion of the exercise The partners recreate the game with a reversed role.

Poon-Sau (Double Sticky Hands)

The 3rd Chi-Sau practice can be described as Poon Sau. It is the first method that is taught to students of Wing-Chun which involves the simultaneous use of both hands. When performing Poon Sau both hands embrace the movement in a circle. For preparation two pupils try to make use of Poon Sau to alter each other's center line.

If they are successful, they'll be able to slay the opponent's defence and use the advantage of their center power, causing them to lose and allowing them to hit. The art of Poon Sau depends on techniques of energy and sensation that are taught in Dan-Chi Sau.

The effectiveness of Poon Sau to defeat any opponent is based on the constantly changing motion, which is able to be a distraction and an attempt to confuse your opponent's mind. While it may sound simple, every hand motion is controlled by carefully controlled adjustments in speed and power. This is a technique that needs time and perseverance to master until it is as natural like breathing.

Luk-Sau (Forward Moving Double Sticky Hands)

Many books on Wing-Chun Kung Fu liken Luk Sau to the prior Poon Sau technique. So, it's the easiest skill to master. Even though the physical elements are the identical, except for one extra however, they will require time and effort to learn. What is new here is how energy will be utilized.

Like Poon Sau, the objective remains to be in control of the partner's center line using the double sticky hand method. But now, it is performed with a forward-facing motion in order in order to execute a winning strike.

Gor-Sau (Free-Technique)

Gor Sau is also begun by taking on that it is based on the Poon Sau structure. Then, each participant moves away from each other and maintains a link by a single arm of their arms. The position that is used in this way is referred to as to be the most basic Gor Sau. Each participant has ample space to work.

This is why the name that is translated as "free technique" develops. Though this can give the two participants an advantage, it can makes it harder for one to identify an opportunity to fend off or overwhelm each other. Since there is no defense both will have be quick to move to keep the other from being aware of their intentions, and reacting by a suitable blocking or counter.

Typical Gradings

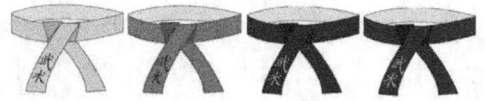

Gradings for all classes differ from one school to the next and, in fact, often differ between each type of Wing-Chun Kung Fu being practiced. These pages offer illustrations of the most popular practices and guidelines to be met for each level within Wing-Chun.

Be aware that colors be different from school to school. For example, a yellow sash in one class could be more prestigious that a yellow sash another. These are the most popular applications of ranking colors.

The grading criteria can be used as an aid to study as a supplement to classes.

Understanding and understanding comes through experience in performing these methods regularly, and acquainting you with their sensations and how they feel, in order to master the techniques with ease and without hesitation should you need to.

Yellow Sash (Grade 1)

The first level of Wing-Chun grade focuses specifically on Siu Lim Tao. To earn this level, a person should demonstrate proficiency in the various forms, as well as excellent knowledge of the basic theories. It is crucial for the beginner to learn this part as almost all hand movements that are used in Wing-Chun can be learnt from Siu Lim Tao. There are several requirements that are placed on beginner in the grade of one.

Students should be able to discuss the various forms within Siu Lim Tao. They should also be able to correctly answer any questions that are asked by them.

Dan-Chi Sau teaches the necessity of performing every position with precision and accurately. The book also explains the different various ways that Wing-Chun's "three seeds' connect to each other.

The Lok-sauor Bong Lap lets the novice to learn foot and handwork at the same time.

Chi-Sau and Gor Sau contains the 10 most basic Wing-Chun skills that the learner must master before moving onto the next level.

Free Hand Techniques comprise the last lesson of Siu Lim Tao. The technique is utilized as an instruction to defend specifically in connection with one strike.

Prerequisites for Yellow Sash:

Perform Siu Lim Tao.

1. Perform your movements with precision and speed.

2. Display a correct form and appropriate use of energy.

3. Explain every move of the figures using proper words.

4. You should be able to demonstrate the method to a instructor or student.

Answer correctly the questions below or follow-up questions.

1. Define the three or four sections in the Siu Lim Tao form in an organized steps-by-step format.

2. What lessons can you take through Siu Lim Tao Form? Siu Lim Tao Form?

Perform Dan-Chi-Sau and/or Lok-Sau.

1. Demonstrate the movements that Dan Chi performs. Dan Chi on each side.

2. Demonstrate Lok-sau.

3. Perform the first 10 Chi-Sau movement.

Chapter 9: Free Hand Techniques

1. Perform all the necessary skills in defending against straight punch. Think about both the inside and the outer gates.

Display knowledge, as well as the capability to debate and use:

1. Wing-Chun Center Line Theory

2. Inner and Outer Gate Theory

3. Three Seeds of Wing-Chun

4. Dan-Chi-Sau

5. Chi-Sau

6. Gor Sau

What ways is Dan-Chi-Sau and BongLap Chi-Sau, Dan-Chi-Sau, and Gor Sau related to each other? Discuss the ways in which they can be utilized separately and in combination.

Green Sash (Grade 2)

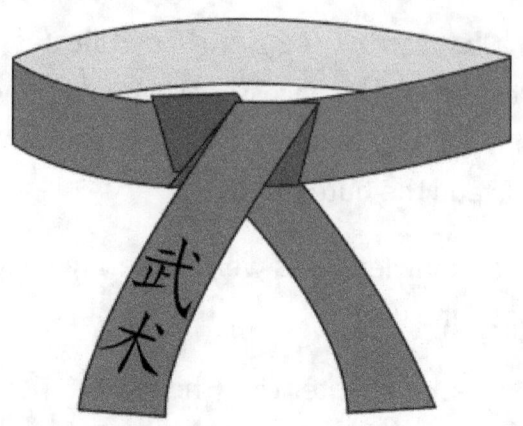

The second grade of Wing-Chun's curriculum will require the student to show the foundation of Chum-Kiu in concrete. When the physical movements are learned, a novice is guided by a deeper and more detailed training course for multidirectional attack and defense techniques.

Students should be capable of analyzing each form or the Chum-Kiu principle and respond to any questions that are they are asked.

How to maintain your balance and perform the footwork. Learn the benefits of the four-distances.

What happened to Lok-sau's development as a result of Bong Sau and how the addition of footwork allows this role to be more adaptable.

Show familiarity with Sau as well as Gor Sau and Gor Sau, including the way they came to be and demonstrate the correct performance of higher level abilities and sequences.

Know the development of Freehand Techniques that are not included in the above list. Learn how to respond to numerous attempts to strike through various blocks. Be aware that the initial strike is most crucial when it comes to a correct reaction.

Identify improvements in the distribution of weight, balance and maintain the center line by demonstrating correct postures.

Prerequisites for Green Sash:

Completion of the entire Chum-Kiu sequence.

1. You can move with precision and ease.

2. Show accurate and correct utilization of energy.

3. Explain every move of the form using the proper words.

4. Learn the forms to a different student or teacher.

Answer correctly the questions below or follow-up questions.

1. Define the three or four parts in the Siu Lim Tao form in an easy steps-by-step format.

2. What is the lesson that Chum-Kiu can teach?

Dan-Chi-Sau/ Lok-sau

1. Perform the moves from Dan Chi.

2. Implement Lok-sau, including the additional footwork.

3. Display progress in their practice of Chi-Sau starting from the first evaluation in terms of speed and response, correct relaxation as well as smoothness, footwork and a variety.

Free Hand Technique

To be able to move on to the next level, every pupil must show improvement in their footwork, as well in their ability to master Chi-Sau as well as its associated moves. Also, they must be proficient using a variety of strike techniques that could be applied against pads to increase their speed and precision when compared to the beginning grade.

Have a basic understanding of the subject and have the ability to talk about:

1. The Bodily-structure theory

2. Chi Gerk

3. The Low-line Kick Theoretical

4. The theory of defense that is multi-direction

5. Multi Directional Offensive Movement Theory

6. The Center Line

7. The Inner and Outer Gates

8. The Four Distance Principle

Brown Sash (Grade 3)

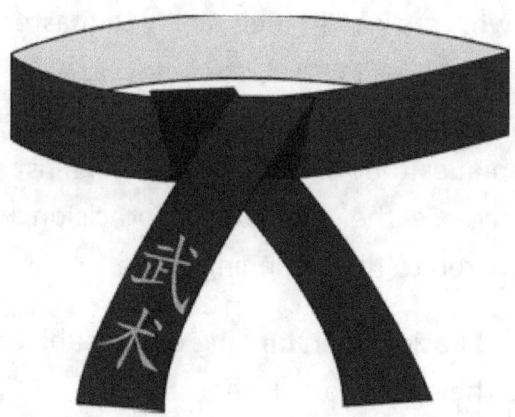

The next level for Wing-Chun is third grade. This is based on a thorough knowledge the concept of Biu Tze. Students will need be able to develop their abilities for keeping their center line.

The student must demonstrate competence with the Biu Tze forms as well as an knowledge of the philosophy employed.

1. Lok-sau continues develop by putting in more footwork as well as better information.

2. Chi-Sau as well as Gor Sau develop through sophisticated techniques and patterns, with and the main goal is to influence opponents into making mistakes, thus giving them the opportunity to strike. The theory of recovery are also important to know in this moment.

3. Free Hand Techniques may be employed against a variety of strikes.

Prerequisites for Brown Sash:

Showcase Biu Tze's completeness.

1. You can move with precision and ease.

2. Show accurate and correct utilization of energy.

3. Explain every move of the figures using proper terminology.

4. Learn the forms to other students or a teacher.

Completely answer these inquiries or prompts

1. Define the three or four parts in the Siu Lim Tao form in detail in a in a step-by-step manner.

2. What could Biu Tze learn?

Explain a range of strategies to protect yourself from:

1. A Direct Punch (Inner and Outer Gates)

2. A Hook Punch.

3. A Straight Kick (Inner and Outer Gates)

Show your skill when switching between gates, from one to another and then returning.

Show how you can effectively utilize blocks.

Learn how to effectively maintain the center line through every move.

Chi-Sau in the presence of:

1. Proper Footwork and Structure

2. Smooth motions

3. Numerous Chi-Sau and Sau techniques.

4. Proper application of forward energy

5. Relaxation

6. Concentration

7. A capability to provide opportunities to strike at an adversary

Self Defense

It is essential to show a solid defense opposition to numerous attack types from different points of view. The student will be evaluated on the way they respond to:

1. Body Hold from behind

2. Body Hold from Front

3. Head lock on Either Side

4. Half-mount Floor Pin

5. Full-mount Floor Pin

To move to the level of third grade Wing-Chun practitioners will also have to master the aforementioned strikes against pads. Instructors will be looking for the speed and accuracy to improve from the previous assessment.

It is expected that one comprehend and be able to explain or apply the following techniques and theories.

1. The Bodily-structure theory

2. Center Line Theory

3. Chi Gerk

4. Close-Quarter Fighting Ability

5. Low-Line Kicking

6. Multi-Direction Defense Theory

7. Multi-Direction Offence Movement Theory

8. Quick-Release Technique

9. The Inner and Outer Gates

Black Sash (Grade 4)

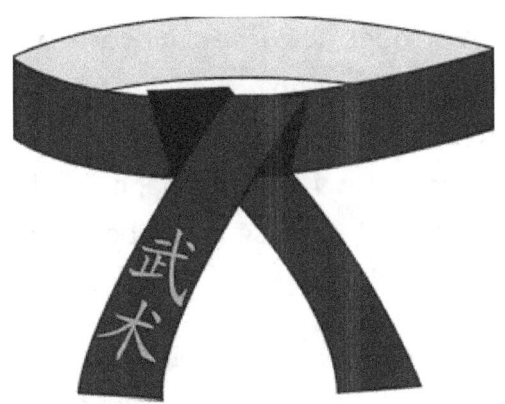

The most advanced stage for Wing-Chun is in the fourth grade. To reach this level, it is necessary for the pupil to master Muk Yan Chong. This could be translated to the "Wooden Dummy Form". Apart from having the ability to perform every form and moves involved and demonstrate knowledge of the various methods and theories that are involved.

The new methods involved when learning the art of Muk Yan Chong includes a range of footwork and hand exercises. It is essential to perform every one of these types and theories when working alongside a friend.

The techniques for free-hand are enlarged upon. In the present, the student must be able to block multiple strikes using a variety of instruments. How they respond to the first strike is crucial because it can be a precursor the whole action.

Students who have completed the fourth grade should demonstrate movement that is exact, smooth and separated well and that effectively use energy.

For the initial time they will learn techniques to increase endurance through correct skeletal alignment.

Prerequisites for Black Sash:

Students must be able to execute Muk Yan Chong by themselves.

1. Display a correct form and appropriate utilization of energy.

2. Explain every move of the figures using suitable words.

3. Learn the forms to a different pupil or an instructor.

The person who is asked to comprehend and talk about the forms that they have already mastered.

1. Biu Tze

2. Chum-Kiu

3. Siu Lim Tao

Free Hand Techniques

At this point, the person who is practicing Wing-Chun must be able to demonstrate every part of the Wooden Dummy Form. They must also be able to break the pattern down into smaller pieces and explaining every part.

They must also show competence in using a variety of defense techniques for defending from high and low-impact attacks within the both inner and outward gates.

The way they execute Free Hand methods. Free Hand methods must exhibit an understanding of how to manage the distance, precise positions that include the use of feet, as well as a proficient utilization of energy.

The student must comprehend and be able to talk about or use the following techniques and theories.

1. Basic close-range fighting skills

2. The Bodily-structure theory

3. Chi Gerk

4. Kicking from the low-line Theoretical

5. Defense theory with multi-direction

6. The theory of multi-direction offenses

7. Quick-release method

8. The Center Line

9. The Inner and Outer Gates

Apart from having an excellent knowledge and skills Fourth-level students must also demonstrate a distinct superiority in comparison to the other students. They must be able to be able to communicate effectively and instruct their classes in both elementary and intermediate levels and concepts.

Chapter 10: Instructors Belt

The top grade level is Instructor. It is only available for students who truly want to become instructors. Sometimes, students who do not wish to instruct will be assessed to determine whether they are able to meet the requirements of an instructor, but they won't be given an upgrade to the level.

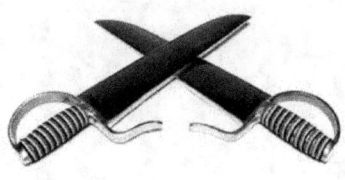

The grade of Wing-Chun is focussed on the use and application of weapons. It is a place where the Butterfly Knife and Pole forms can be used with the highest commitment. For the ability to advance to the instructor's level, practitioners must develop an in-depth understanding of the origins of pole forms and how it was incorporated into the Wing-Chun method. Additionally, they must understand what the intent behind the methods in a situation.

The Pole Techniques

The Sticky Pole Techniques

Long Range Weapon Usage

Prerequisites for Instructors Belt:

Learn and demonstrate proficiency in how to use the Butterfly Knife Form along with various other positions that require advanced skills use of energy, the movements of your feet.

Be proficient in the handling of close and long range guns.

Learn about the advantages as well as the drawbacks to every weapon, including the best feet and space to use the various.

It is important to embody the idea that the knives were designed to be an integral element of the arm. Display the essential premise that all movements can be performed in the same method with no hands.

Discussion of ways how a certain weapon could be effectively used against the various Wing-Chun guns.

Demonstrate understanding of Weapon Attachment Theory.

Understand the techniques that close-range weapons can be utilized.

Becoming a Wing-Chun Instructor

To be able to attain the knowledge of a WingChun instructor, students will require a professional and have a sense of community in the class. That means they must take every class seriously and are willing to help fellow students and their students as much as they can. They also need to be competent in presenting and instructing various methods to fellow Wing-Chun students. Additionally, they must be able to coach individuals and help students in achieving the best results from each technique or technique. In addition, they need be able to develop and carry out an extensive program of instruction.

Prerequisites to Become an Instructor of Wing-Chun

Demonstrate the Eight Slashing Knives (Bart Cham Dao).

1. You can move with precision and ease.

2. Explain every move of the figures using proper words.

3. You should be able to demonstrate the forms to another instructor or student.

4. Learn about Weapon Attachment Theory.

Perform Wooden Pole Form (Luk Dim Boon Kwun).

1. Perform your movements with precision and speed.

2. Define every motion of the figures using proper terminology.

3. You should be able to demonstrate the forms to a different pupil or an instructor.

Demonstrate Wooden Dummy Form (Muk Yan Chong).

1. Perform your movements with precision and speed.

2. Define every motion of the form using the suitable words.

3. You should be able to demonstrate the method to a pupil or an instructor.

Execute the Third Freehand Movement (Biu Tze).

1. Perform your movements with precision and speed.

2. Be sure to breathe properly while you are performing.

3. Explain every move of the form using the proper words.

4. You should be able to demonstrate the forms to another pupil or an instructor.

Perform the Second Freehand Form (Chum-Kiu)

1. Perform your movements with precision and speed.

2. Explain every move of the form using the proper words.

3. You should be able to demonstrate the method to a pupil or an instructor.

Demonstrate the First Freehand Form (Siu Lim Tao)

1. You can move with precision and ease.

2. Explain every move of the form using the suitable words.

3. You should be able to demonstrate the method to a instructor or student.

Apart from having the ability to perform and instruct the steps that are listed in the earlier list students who want to become an instructor needs to be able to discuss these terms on the level of an expert.

Forms:

1. Bart Cham Dao
2. Biu Tze
3. Bong Lap
4. Chi-Sau
5. Chum-Kiu
6. Dan-Chi-Sau
7. Gor Sau
8. Luk Dim Boon Kwun
9. Muk Yan Chong
10. Siu Lim Tao

Theories:

1. Advanced Close Quarter Combat
2. Body Structure
3. Chi Gerk
4. Inner and Outer Gate

5. Multiple Directional Defense

6. Multiple Directional Offensive Movement

7. Low-line kicking

8. Technique for quick-release

9. Weapon Attachment

10. Wing-Chun Center Line

The student who is aspiring to become an instructor must be ready to take part in multiple classes so that they can build on their skills in Wing-Chun as well as continue to develop.

Chapter 11: Wing Chun?

Wing Chun is regarded as one of the most well-known and admired forms of kung fu that come out of Southern China. Contrary to the expansive, broad circular and sometimes acrobatic actions that are often found in kung fu of Northern China (and seen in numerous films) Wing Chun is more gentle, straightforward and linear, promoting an idea of "economy of movement" as well as "no wasted motion." Since it has an lack of circular motions as well as flashy kicks and complex acrobatics It's a great martial art that is suitable for anyone of any age as well as level of physical fitness.

One of the main reason why Southern Chinese martial arts such like Wing Chun evolved so differently in comparison to the Northern Chinese counterparts is due to the environment. The environment in Southern China there was many close-knit communities that had narrow streets and alleyways away from the vast, sprawling countrysides that are found in the North.

Due to this, styles from the south like Wing Chun became more street-oriented and focused on narrow stances, with fast, quick bursts strength. That's why Wing Chun is often known as one of the earliest authentic "street fight" martial arts. It can also make it one of the most effective to use in everyday self-defense.

Another feature that is unique to Wing Chun is its focus to end fights swiftly by making use of fast "chain punching" methods Eye jabs, strikes for the groin and throat striking knee joints as well as striking with clinches. Through educating students on how important it is to rapidly close the gap on their adversary using "forward intention" it isn't a lot of moving around or fancy footwork that you observe with a boxer or kickboxer. The aim of martial arts is to get your job completed quickly and efficiently, using as little effort energy, effort, or wasteful movement as you can making sure that battles get resolved promptly.

Because of this non-committal style, Wing Chun is not an actual fighting sport however it's a swift and deadly street style that is able to do anything so long as it is able to win the match.

One of the most well-known practitioners who practiced Wing Chun was the legendary martial artist Bruce Lee who trained under the famed master Ip Man (portrayed in the film by actor Donnie Yen in the film Ip Man) at Hong Kong. The fundamentals of movements, philosophy, and movements of Wing Chun that comprised the majority of Bruce Lee's distinctive form in Jeet Kun Do.

WHO INVENTED WING CHUN AND WHAT IS ITS HISTORY?

Since the story of Wing Chun was passed down by word of mouth rather than written it is not a reliable basis for its origin, and there are numerous conflicting stories about the person who created it and what inspired its creation. The theory is that some myths are fabricated to conceal the truth about the history that are behind Wing Chun during times of conflict and war, during the period when Shaolin temples were destroyed and a lot of martial artists were viewed as rebels.

One of the most well-known and popular legends about the history of Wing Chun's birth is that about Ng Mui and Yim Wing Chun. The story tells how an Abbess female from Ng Mui's Fujian Shaolin Monastery named Ng Mui managed to escape devastation of the Temple by Qing forces and fled to the vast wilderness of the Daliang Mountains (on the border of Yunnan in China and Sichuan).

In hiding, she discovered a fight between the snake and an unidentified white crane. As she watched the battle, she was able to see the different variations of the styles used by the dashing and darting of the snake against weaving and bobbing skills from the crane.

In the aftermath of watching the fight Ng Mui merged the lessons she had learned along with the years of Shaolin Kung-Fu instruction to develop a completely modern fashion.

In this time Ng Mui used to often deliver bean curd to the store of a lady named Yim Yee who was the mother of an infant daughter called Yim Wing Chun.

Yim Wing Chun is gorgeous, and the local warlord tried to pressure her into marriage.

Ng Mui was inspired to instruct Yim Wing Chun her new combat style, and immediately employed it to defeat the lord of war.

Then, Yim Wing Chun married the person she loved, Leung Bok-Chao. They Leung Bok-Chao taught her the way to dress and even named the system in her honor"Wing Chun" Wing Chun or "eternal springtime."

There are many versions of the same tale, such as one story in which Yim Wing Chun fought a warlord who tried to force her into wedding to a fight. The question was, if she beat him, she would not need to get married. Once she had defeated him using her unique style of kung-fu She got married to the person she loved.

In spite of the fact that the tales are real or which story is true, the same aspects always play a role such as the observation of the snake as well as the crane combat, along with the way of fighting developed by a woman. This illustrates the way Wing Chun is able to beat bigger strong opponents using only a little strength.

The image of the snake and crane is also crucial for Wing Chun because it is a symbol of several hand movements. For instance, poking and darting movements in Biu Sao (representative of the snake striking) as well as the techniques of covering and diverting including Fuk Sao (representative for the crane).

One of the interesting aspects of the story of Wing Chun is how it was adopted by the Red Boat Opera Company as an obscure style that was only taught by those who are within "the well-informed." In the Red Boat Opera

Company was one of the groups consisting of Chinese touring opera singers that traveled throughout China during the latter part of 1800 to the early 1900s.

There is a popular belief it is possible that Red Boat Opera Company was in fact a disguise of Qing Dynasty rebels who would cover their martial arts instruction to disguise themselves as stage tricks to improve their abilities to defeat the army troops.

It was Ip Man who first began to teach Wing Chun openly in the 1950s in Hong Kong, which allowed ordinary people (like Bruce Lee) to study the martial art, and then spread it across all over the world.

WHEN IS A GOOD TIME TO START WING CHUN?

There's never a time more appropriate than now. It's not necessary to wait until you've achieved a certain amount of fitness or strength. Since Wing Chun is just as appropriate for young people as it is for people of a certain age, you'll enjoy the benefits of starting Wing Chun no matter where you're in your journey.

WILL I BE OUT OF PLACE?

If you go to class you will meet students who are smarter than you do. So don't be concerned about that. We are aware that our Wing Chun students and teachers are part of a family. Everyone who puts food on the kitchen is a member of our family too.

If you've had previous experience in martial arts or if the most strenuous exercise you've ever done was to climb the stairs up to get into your home - you'll fit just right in an environment that is completely free of judgement.

We aim to make you feel at ease, assist you, and aid you in understanding the principles and techniques of Wing Chun so that you are able to apply the physical exercises and principles to your own life.

There's a phrase that is used in Wing Chun circles, "Wing Chun is not visible and must be experienced." Since Wing Chun is very subtle with no flashy motions, it could be difficult for anyone who is just watching to grasp what's taking place since Wing Chun often LOOKS as even though there's nothing happening.

This is why it's crucial to be able to feel Wing Chun - to understand the impact it can have upon your body after being it is used and when you're practicing it.

We aren't allowing people to observe a class. We rather encourage potential or new students to join us during"open days" or "open day" for a class with other students who work with you to explain the basics.

IS WING CHUN SUITABLE FOR EVERYONE?

No matter if you're old, young overweight, slim, female, or male Wing Chun is perfect for you. Actually, of the many traditional martial arts ranging that range from Karate and Jiu Jitsu - Wing Chun is most likely the one that's least physical demanding. This is an aspect of the appeal of the martial art that has been practiced for centuries. It is just as efficient swift, dangerous, and deadly regardless of the physical condition. A person who is able to run 5 miles with no fatigue and an overweight person with a back injury will have the ability to use the same strategies to the same effect.

IS WING CHUN SUITABLE FOR THE DISABLED?

In short, it's dependent on the type of disability. There are plenty of instances where people who are blind, suffer from cerebral palsy, who have a disability that requires wheelchairs, or are suffering from various disabilities can successfully practice Wing Chun in their own method. Since Wing Chun is not physically demanding and extremely adaptable, it's safe to state that there is a vast range of disabilities that are able to get the most benefits from learning Wing Chun.

Please let us know in advance whether you are suffering from a specific handicap. We'll do our best to meet your needs.

AM I TOO OLD FOR WING CHUN?

If you're still able to be able to drive, eat or make your bed and go shopping, it's not too late to learn Wing Chun. One of the benefits to Wing Chun is how seamlessly it evolves as we age. Anyone who starts training as a teenager will be able to work as intensely and have the same ability in their 80s. In accordance with the concept of "no wasted movements" when it comes to Wing Chun, strikes and methods do not depend on strength of muscles, physical acceleration, or aerobic feetwork. Instead, it is based on being able to apply the most force to achieve the greatest amount of force. As a result, you will spend more time practicing how to let go and not depend on physical strength or capability in Wing Chun, which makes the perfect choice for those who are older.

WHAT ARE THE REQUIREMENTS FOR TRAINING WING CHUN?

Don't let your self-esteem go to the door. Don't treat your life too seriously, let you to fail but be willing and determined to learn new techniques. Like all skills in life practicing is necessary and put in the time and be constant in your efforts to master.

But, if you're having difficulties time learning, feel you have more knowledge than instructors, or your primary intention is to be in physical combat, it's better not to train Wing Chun.

Chapter 12: What Does A Typical Class Consist Of?

The typical class begins with a light workout and stretching exercises to warm up your body. Following that, we might begin by introducing the first form of Wing Chun (Sil Lum Tao), practice a few kick and punching drills or even work on pad drills in conjunction with your partner.

Every class is focused on hands-on activities and a partnership. Our instructors pair students according to their level of skill and typically spend the greater part of the class learning a particular skill using a range of techniques to "drill" the method into your head, practice it and then ensure that the technique becomes second-nature.

DO YOU HAVE A GRADING SYSTEM?

While traditional kung fu did not have no grade system however, we've discovered it is essential to separate students based on their experience in Wing Chun. But, it shouldn't be the intention of students to move up the grades in order to earn the recognition that comes with the process. This is why we do not place a lot of importance on rapid progression through our system of grading, and don't believe that our students ought to either.

The students progress through the system of grading based on the knowledge they have of Wing Chun's fundamentals the philosophy, techniques, and principles. As an example, anyone could learn to do the moves in Sil Lum Tao. Sil Lum Tao form, but are they aware of the purpose of these movements? Are they able to channel energy into these motions? Do they know the name of every movement, and describe the purpose behind it?

To learn more about our system of grading, to a class, and speak to any of our coaches.

DO I NEED TO BE AGGRESSIVE?

No matter if you are an aggressive individual or think you are a passive individual The primary purpose in Wing Chun is to get your mind relaxed and to comprehend the movements from both an intellectual and technical perspective, and to develop you from the bottom upwards.

Once you've done that, you'll learn how to handle aggression, and also what degrees of aggressiveness are required in a particular circumstance - beginning with training sessions that are friendly with a friend to street fight.

When you first learn to manage your own actions, as well as your thoughts and body, you'll be able to employ physical violence whenever needed.

But, in the event that we exercise our minds, the aim isn't aggression, and, if you think of yourself as an individual who is not prone to conflicts, you won't be overwhelmed by the desire to display an aggressive character in the absence of one.

WILL I GET HURT IN CLASS?

When you engage in any kind of physical exercise, there's a chance of injury The same goes when driving a vehicle or jogging along the streets. But, unlike entering an ring for boxing in which it is possible to be subjected to punches to your face or the body, this doesn't be the case when you practice Wing Chun. While sparring is a possibility however, it's managed and full-contact is reserved for those who have mastered their attacks and who are training in Wing Chun for an extended time time.

The Wing Chun system does put the emphasis on strengthening and enhancing the forearms, knuckles, palms, and fingers by hitting hard surfaces like bags that are filled with beans and buckets filled with sand, or wooden dolls (Mook Jong). It will eventually result in bleeding. It is important to do the process slowly, forming the bones slowly over time. Thus, while you might be prone to bruises, it are not likely to suffer some kind of serious injury.

DO I HAVE TO BE FIT TO START?

Absolutely no. Training regimens like those within Wing Chun will undoubtedly improve the level of fitness up to a certain degree however that's not an indication that the training itself is difficult or exhausting. Apart from a few light workouts in the first part of every class, along with some small-scale pad work and sparring Wing Chun training itself does need a lot of physical or flexibility. There is no need to sling high kicks as well as jumping and running.

Since Wing Chun stresses economy of movements and having no wasted motion The goal is to use as much force as you can with the smallest amount of effort. As a result, Wing Chun is more concentrated on calming the mind and body and gaining the ability to make rapid, quick, and explosive shot rather than intricate, intense cardio exercises.

HOW LONG WILL IT TAKE TO GET GOOD?

It all is entirely dependent on the individual degree of attendance and commitment, your ability to comprehend the more profound concepts and the philosophies behind the method, how much time you spend practicing in your spare time as well as other factors.

But, it's safe to state that when they attend regularly an average student will have the ability to employ an array of methods correctly and proficiently in 6 months of education.

This Wing Chun system itself was created to be a quick and easy learning system. Instead of having numerous types (such in other systems, such as Choy Lee Fut or Northern Shaolin) Wing Chun only offers three hands, three open forms, a wooden dummy as well as two forms of weapons to make a total of 6.

Although, even though the methods used in Wing Chun are simple and straightforward does not necessarily mean that there's no other layers. While a person can be taught how to properly apply techniques in just six months, understanding the meaning behind movement and learning how to swiftly respond to sudden situations as well as honeing the sensitivity of skills like Chi Sao and Lop Sao can take much longer time.

WHAT ARE THE WING CHUN FORMS

As opposed to traditional martial art like Japanese Karate's Katas and sometimes the hundreds of forms that are found in the popular Chinese Kung fu forms, Wing Chun keeps it very straightforward. Three empty hand types and one dummy made of wood as well as two forms for weapons.

While Wing Chun not have a vast number of styles but the forms that the system does offer are simple straightforward, basic and do not require huge movements that are sweeping. Indeed, the most fundamental of all the forms in the Wing Chun system (Sil Lum Tao) is totally stationary and requires absolutely no footwork.

The most effective method to conceptualize the forms of Wing Chun is to view the forms as the "catalogue" of moves. In this way, ALL martial arts come with forms. For example, in boxing using the technique that is known as "shadow boxing" is one of the activities that boxers commonly take part in. It is a way for them to warm up, test their technique, and practice in the absence of bags or teammates to work using. Shadow boxing is easy It allows the boxer to use the standard movement of the foot, bobbing weave and also the most basic punches in boxing (jab or hook, cross and uppercut).

Similar to how a boxer, Muay Thai practitioner, or grappler would train in the basics of their discipline in a single space, the Wing Chun practitioner will practice our movements in a solitary environment. This is done in order to "drill" the fundamental techniques of the system the solitude of our own environment for a variety of reasons.

To make sure that the movement becomes second nature

To consider each step separately as part of an overall

To keep in mind the goal of each move

A free-flowing meditation sensation

Once you know the reasons how important forms are to Wing Chun, let's look at the 6 forms in the System.

Chapter 13: Empty Hand Wing Chun Forms

Sil Lum Tao (Little Idea)

Though it's not the simplest Wing Chun form - as it's static and doesn't require any steps - Sil Lum Tao remains considered to be the most significant Wing Chun form as it symbolizes what is known as the Wing Chun philosophy and the entirety of the system's base.

From the outside Sil Lum Tao appears to be nothing special. But the significance of this design can't be overstated. It is a quick form and take 2 minutes or less but it could also be a long one, that takes 20 or more minutes. It may be little other than a basic form to master Wing Chun's basic hands, stances, and centerline concept and can also be more of a deep and meditative exercise (Qigong) where one slows down, controlling the breath, and then transferring one's energy into the earth as an exercise that is known as "rooting."

In the form itself, you learn fundamental hand movements such Tan Sau (dispersing hand),

Fook Sau (covering/prostrating hand), Wu Sau (protecting hand), Pak Sau (slapping hand), and more.

Since the posture is stationary and slack, it trains your posture, enhancing your legs as well as improving your ability to balance.

Chum Kiu (Bridging The Gap / Seeking The Bridge)

It is the second variant of Wing Chun. In contrast to Sil Lum Tao, Chum Kiu does not rely on a single hand to perform. In contrast to Sil Lum Tao where most methods are performed using just only one hand at time, Chum Kiu gets two hands working in tandem (along with movement that the foot makes). Chum Kiu also employs some simple moves (snap and kicks).

The purpose to Chum Kiu with regards to "bridging gaps" is to teach you to close quickly the distance between yourself and your adversary, thereby disrupting their physical structure, and then throw off balance by using various close-range techniques including elbows, knees and elbows employed to perform Wing Chun.

Biu Ji (Thrusting Fingers / Little Finger Pointing to The Moon)

If you can recall one of the major issues surrounding the creation of the form of Wing Chun, in which Ng Mui was the person who claimed to be the creator saw a snake and crane fighting in the woods and thought of that Biu Ji form and its strategies as the fangs that strike that the snake.

Biu Ji employs a number of the most dangerous open-hand techniques used within Wing Chun, namely the "stabbing fingers" which target the areas that are most susceptible to attack people, like their eyes as well as their neck. It is possible to imagine changing your hand to a sword or needle and swiftly and firmly attack.

Biu Ji consists of both long and short range strategies, complete with sweeps and low kicks. The form is a way to teach elbow strikes as well as recovering from circumstances where the opponent has lost their "center line" in a fight.

There's a famous Wing Chun saying, "Biu Ji isn't going out the front door." In most cases, this is understood as meaning that the method is to be kept under wraps or should not be utilized unless you are able to assist to prevent it from being used. These techniques are intended meant to cause death and injury particularly when one is studying how to use pressure points.

Wing Chun WOODEN Dummy FormThe Mook Jong also known as "Wooden Dummy" is an essential form of training in different forms of Kung Fu, especially Wing Chun. While there's only one wooden dummy used in Wing Chun, it has many movements, and it is very intricate.

The wooden dummy mimics the human body (which is the reason it's often known as a wooden man) that has two arms stretched out with one hand located in the middle (mimicking punching low) as well as a curving "foot" in the lower part that allows leg kicks.

One of the primary reasons for the wooden dummy shape is training the performer to be mobile and attack and move about the adversary while also defense, by using deft movements, kicks and footwork moving with angularity without losing an arc of center.

The Wooden Dummy brings together all three empty hand designs and then applies these to the real world of an adversary where the force you strike will be met with real resist.

Another important element of training with wooden dummies is the conditioning of body, or "iron body" methods. Through hitting the Dummy for a long period of time in varying levels of force, begin to see your bones develop tiny hairline fractures. As your bones heal, they will get stronger, allowing you to strike the wooden dummy more forcefully and harder with no discomfort.

If you practice on the wooden dummy, you develop your knuckles palms, and forearms making your arms an instrument. After a couple of months of practicing with the wooden model, your hands, palms and forearms will grow more durable as well as "sharper." Hitting people with knuckles in conditionally suited is different from hitting them with knuckles which don't. It doesn't just hurt the person being attacked more (because you've conditioned your arms and hands) it also hurts the person you are aiming at significantly.

WING CHUN WEAPON FORMS

In keeping with the current trend of simplicity in The Wing Chun system, there only two weapons taught in the Wing Chun system namely, the butterfly knives and dragon pole (staff). It is not like other Chinese kung-fu styles which utilize a broader selection of training with weapons (spears as well as long swords, broad swords, as well as various variations of the tools) Wing Chun only concentrates on two weapons.

Today, a lot of people find no reason to learning something such as butterfly knives, or even long poles. In the end, who's likely to carry around two massive knives or an eight to thirteen foot long pole any time? What are these things going to be in the vicinity when people are attacking you in the streets?

In this case, what's the purpose of the training?

However, it is highly unlikely that anyone carried butterflies or long poles all over the place at the time Wing Chun was invented and teaching it secretly is highly unlikely.

The reasons these two weapon types are used has nothing to do of whether they could (or should) really be utilized in a regular basis.

Their training method is more practical than what we'll take a look at in the next section.

Baat Jam Dao - Wing Chun Btterfly Swords (Eight Cut Swords)

One of the best things with Butterfly Swords is how utterly different they can be. They may be utilized for slashing at enemies however, the reverses of the blades may also be utilized to slash, crush, fracture, or block attacks with a slash, as an example, striking the wrist. In the past, butterfly swords were commonly referred to by the name of Dit Ming Do (Life-taking knives).

The purpose in this Batt Jam Dao form, apart from showing the different parrying, slashing and stabbing actions you are able to employ with your knives is to let the knives to be the extension that extends your arm.

Actually. You will be accustomed to using your empty hand when carrying weapons. It prepares you for using many different weapons including knives and short sticks but without sacrificing the efficiency and fundamentals of the empty hand technique.

When you get used to knives as extensions from your hands, you are able to change them out with a variety of different objects.

Look Dim Boon Grun (Dragon Pole / Six and Half Point Pole)

In the past I'm able to think of a handful of situations where you could have access to a rod anywhere between 5 to 13 feet in length at any time. Then, what's the significance of the dragon pole?

To begin consider this: think of a pole, which is about one inch wide. The pole becomes very heavy.

It's advantageous the way it improves grip, wrists and also your arms. Also, it improves the strength of your "driving force" that is the capability to rapidly explode forward by utilizing a tremendous, explosive force.

The practice of the dragon pole, in The Look Dim Boon Grun form significantly increases your stamina, strength grip, as well as powerful footwork. This can be translated directly into free-hand Wing Chun techniques.

Chapter 14: Wing Chun Techniques

Like we said earlier, Wing Chun is a traditional Southern Chinese martial art, which originated within the Shao Lin Monastery in the "Spring Temple" and hence, the term Wing Chun means Forever Spring. As opposed to other forms which focus more on the retraining of an opponent as well as decreasing the amount of damage down to the lowest level.

The basic concept is built upon three elements:

1. Facing. If someone is practicing the method in a fight it is best to make the whole body look in towards the in the same direction. This is known as "facing" because it indicates that your body isn't turning about. Face-to-face can assist the user to be more focused while using the entire body to its maximum. If facing properly the face can be positioned in an ideal position to strike.

2. Center line. This means that from the highest point of his head down to the bottom

of his foot the line is formed. One should aim with his center line until the the centerline of his opponent, since that is the closest distance between them. If both fighters strike at similar speed of strike, the closer the distance is, the higher chance to strike the goal.

3. Straight. The reason a person has to be straight is because they can unleash their energy more efficiently and quickly.

Because the idea is just as crucial as the method employing the right concept in conjunction with being mindful of all the body's posture can help create the body to be flexible.

Wing Chun technique consists of three forms of hands:

1. Xiu Lim Tao, also known as Little Idea.

2. Chum Kiu, also called Chrom Kiu is also known as Seeking.

3. Biu Jee, also called Thrusting Fingers.

To Xiu Lim Tao, there are various hand movements that are defensive in nature.

The second one is Tan Sau that means Dispersing Hand. Tan Sau is among the three foundations of Wing Chun techniques (Tan Sau, Bong Sau, Fook Sau). The first method to be taught in the Wing Chun Character Sun Fist as well as the best method to incorporate with other methods. To some extent, Tan Sau means loosening hand. In Wing Chun, Tan Sau is the term used to allow your hand of the opponent diverge from the center line with your arm so that you can release the force. The technique requires your entire arm. Likewise, your wrist must remain straight. A curve of any kind could cause injury to yourself. It's mostly used for directing or stop the flow of force after meeting the force. In order to perform this method it is recommended that the user put on his elbows. Tan Sau is a method that is passive and not active, as it can be altered depending on the strike of the opponent's modifications.

The Tan Sau technique can be executed in the following manner:

1. Open to Yee Gee Kim Yeung Ma (this will be mentioned near the close of article).

2. Fist turns into palm;

3. Develop the strength from the tip of the elbow and finger. remove the palm from the body's center line. Keep the heart of your palm up while the palm remains sitting in supine.

Instructional Video of Wing Chun Tan Sau:

A Demonstration Video of Tan Sau and Wooden Dummy Training:

The other name is Huen Sau which means Circling Hand. This is an effective method to focus on wrist movements. It is a great technique to take on the strength of the opponent, and also to shift the direction of your wrist between outside and inside or even from inside to outside. Tan Sau as well as Huen Sau are able to be used along with different techniques. The general rule is that after finishing each move, the technique will be transferred into Huen Sau or Wu Sau to conclude.

How to do Hauen Sau:

Following Huen Sau, hands are drawn inwards, which is known as Wu Sau. This is sometimes referred to as the Guarding Hand. In this manner one puts his or her hand on their elbows and draws all the strength from the wrist.

How to do Wu Sau:

The second option is Fook Sau; it means subduing hand. This is typically utilized to regulate your own place in the fight in the event of a bridge being constructed. In general, when your the palm's heart is downwards either forward or to the right or left, it will be Fook Sau. As you hold Fook Sau without moving the body, it will feel like the muscles in your chest and armpits are relaxing. If the exterior of your arms, your back your body and legs feel stretched and tight, this is one of the methods to generate power, and could affect the result.

How to Do Fook Sau:

The other option refers to Pak Sau, which means Slapping Hand. The hand is slapped in the middle, while the elbow and wrist at the all time move toward the chest. If two people engage in a fight the aim is to knock the other person out. There are two methods to increase the power of Wing Chun: Long Bridge and Short Bridge, and Bridge is a reference towards the forearm. This is Long Bridge when elbow is expanding, and Short Bridge when elbow is curving. Pak Sau is in the area in the range of Short Bridge for defence.

How to do Pak Sau:

There are other hand forms that are defensive in 2. Chum Kiu and its strike techniques include Gum Sau and between middle and up Bong Sau along with various moves and kicks.

Gum Sau means Pressing Hand. This is the process of pushing hands downwards.

How to do Gum Sau:

Bong Sau refers to Bong Sau is a reference to Wing Arm Bong Sau is one of the most significant and flexible methods. The idea is to utilize your body's structure at different angles, with different directions and through rotations to produce power. This will result in dealing with hardness while being soft, as well as making use of the force of your opponent in order to increase your advantages. It will help you alter the direction that your opponent strikes from. Its role is to make advantage of your body's structure in order to squelch the attack from the front. Girls can also withstand an opponent's powerful fist making use of Bong Sau when she is able to master this method because it allows her to shift between short distance and long distance, or between defence and strike in the course of a fight.

How to Do Bong Sau aka Wing Hand:

The second Chi Sau is also known as sticking hand. It's used to instruct students to observe the flow of force of the other's hands and following their hand movements. In this process it is not necessary to increase speed, just to keep following in a concordance. If you are performing this exercise be sure to ensure the hands and front arms are submissive, but not weak, and dynamically however not rigid. at the same time, make sure that the center line does not start shifting.

How to do Chi Sau:

Biu Sau, commonly referred to by the name of Thrusting Fingers is a part of the highest level of striking that are used in Wing Chun techniques. It's the technique of hitting that has a radical change to the old technique, inherited from and advancing methods like Siu Lim Tao and Chum Kiu. This method requires hitting in order to push small power against massive power by borrowing power from the entire body. Biu Sau is always used to determine if the opponent is more powerful than you are. Biu Sau can be utilized to strike your opponent's weak areas like eyes or neck using fingers. The fingers must be locked and most important is that wrists must remain straight and secure. If this method is used then the wrist must be robust. It is basically how you can generate explosive force using your body's parts that could be fingers palms, fists and palms elbows and arms. The general rule is that Biu Sau refers to an Wing Chun technique which includes intermediate, short and long distance strikes.

How to do Biu Sau:

The distinction between Thrusting Hand and Thrusting Finger isn't huge. Thrusting Hand can be utilized to deal with straight line or curvature line attacks. In the first place, it could be employed to protect the internal gate. In addition, it blocks the attacker's hand so that it is prevented from contacting any part of his body before he finishes his blow. It is one of the best techniques to manage area.

Elbows are used in techniques for short range. The ideal attack location is the back and surface portion. To generate the power to explode, it is necessary to focus on the shoulder line. You can also attempt to utilize other areas of the body, e.g. rotating the hips in order to bring the shoulder line back towards the middle. The power of the elbow that causes injury originates from the hip.

There is a second idea referred to as "Emergency Hand". When you are in combat it is not always according to plan, and what seems like one of the most basic things could be the hardest thing to do. The emergency Hand technique is a great way to get back to health, and it's an innovative element of Biu Sau, which can assist your body to return in a more balanced position. Because Wing Chun is a defensive practice, if someone is holding your hand, they will stop your attack, and when you are in this position, you could make use of Pressing Elbow to get back control of your opponent. The primary targets for elbows are faces, head and arms. The strike could come from a variety of directions, including from the sides or back. It is as well as from the front. The strike could be diagonal, horizontal as well as vertical. The advantage is of using your elbows to safeguard yourself from different angles. The purpose of this method is to adapt and change.

Wing Chun techniques focus on the area in front of the body. When two people are in contact, the first thing to employ is the Asking Hand (sometimes known as the Sending Off Hand). When you're standing in the middle with someone else in front of you, you've no idea from where the attacker comes from or the area that the person is getting hit. However, when you sense that there's something moving towards the gate in your upper direction, you could reach out your arms and hands quickly and forcefully to block your gate. However, you should not reaching out your hands as if you were touching anything, and if you do it quickly, as it could become explosive.

The following idea is the Long Bridge Grasping Hand. This is more than just grasping hand, but it should be swift and explosive. This isn't just exclusive to hands; it can also involve the arm and head. It is about keeping enough space to strike. The posture will ensure your safety and security, therefore it's the technique of control, which can lead you to the next stage -- the strike technique which is that is, the Ginger Punch, to hit those areas that are sensitive to the body.

One of the most famous striking methods is Lin Wan Keun, the chain punch. The name suggests that you know it's a continuous strike, that is extremely robust. By using the power of your elbow and straight line, hitting repeatedly it is possible to put your opponent in a place without strength against you. This technique has become popular as the best example of the Wing Chun fist technique. The most important aspect in this technique is to maintain a relaxed fist and hold it tight until the time of striking, keep the fist to be in an even line when striking and striking in the same way continuously. ensure that shoulders are in a balanced position as well as lock the fist, wrist, and front arm within the same straight direction.

What is the Lin Wan Kun (AKA "the chain punch)

In addition, One Inch Punch also has a significant place in the Wing Chun fist system. The one inch distance is very short and as the title suggests, and so requires the player to aim to achieve the highest force at a small distance. One of the most important aspects to manage effectively is to take advantage of the chance for acceleration. The ideal time to increase speed occurs when the tense punch is able to touch the skin (garment) and at the time at the same time the punch is released with the strongest force. One inch of punch is an art that is a way to learn and practice both in both external and internal. While it may appear to be a simple, ordinary however, it is an extremely fatal strike. The most powerful Wing Chun fighter has the capability to break through the box completely in about 1-3 inches in a short distance.

Explaination of the one-inch punch:

The introductions in the previous paragraphs are upper body movements, so here are the fundamental technique called Yee Jee Kim Yeung Ma. This is the most fundamental posture that is performed at the bottom of your body. The term Ma is a horse word, and originates from the old cavalryman who rode the war horse. An excellent solider must always be a part of the horse overall. Yee Jee signifies that when the heel and toe form an Chinese symbol "Er " The distance between the toes needs to be slightly less than between heels. The gesture is able to provide powerful adhering power to the feet when it is placed on the ground. If you do Yee Jee Kim Yeung Ma properly The barycenter should sit approximately 1 inch behind the feet center. In between, body weight must be divided between both the sides of the barycenter. Additionally, the upper body must face toward the center. The waist should be straight.

Yee Jee Kim Yeung Ma:

Wing Chun, as a as a whole, is a defensive method that focuses on helping your body to release energy and return the body's center line to maintain control over space. Each move is impressive and extremely explosive. The premise behind Wing Chun is very efficient particularly in close-range combat. The principle of guarding is to utilize a minimum amount of time and energy as well as minimal body movement, for the greatest protection.

Chapter 15: The 3 Non-Negotiable Elements

The reasons for injuries vary but I'm not taking the time to go through every possibility, since it would be impossible. Instead, I'd like concentrate on three aspects which must be balanced in order to reduce the risk of injury that can cause injury: mobility, flexibility and the strength. These three characteristics constitute the base for any person who wants to improve their athletic performance starting from the 70-year-old grandmother to the athlete who is 22. They form the basis that will help you achieve your chances of success. When any of these three elements is not in balance the result is an ideal environment for injury to happen.

Let's begin with the most straightforward aspect to consider the strength issue. It is an incredibly simple ability to acquire. The basic fitness and strength program that you follow every week for a few times under the supervision by a qualified professional will increase your strength in a short time, particularly those who already play an activity that encourages development of the strength.

The other element is mobility. It can be defined as the capability to move a limb joint in a full movement range with the help of a. The work of mobility is a voluntary one and requires strength in order to complete the task (flexibility is typically a active skill, requiring static holding to stretch the muscles of the body). Mobility and flexibility are essential skills for an sportsperson to be able to master However, their development of these abilities is not often considered when the training process. The more mobile a person is, the more quickly and easily they will be able to complete their task. It doesn't matter if it's making a roundhouse kick, passing guard, or buying a box of food, more mobility is always a sign of improved effectiveness.

Each person will experience unique issues with mobility. For a successful treatment you must talk to a doctor and then be educated on the best way to manage your particular condition. The most frequent conditions I observe often in the gym are an impingement in the hips as well as shoulders. A lot of martial arts put a heavy demands on these joints as well as their muscles surrounding them.

An excellent way to boost mobility is by using myofascial releases and various other exercises that are designed specifically to improve the proper motion of the limb or joint. There are two strategies to improve the flexibility of your shoulder and hips.

Myofascial release of the shoulder Girdle

Begin lying on your back using a foam roller on your hip. Begin to slowly roll upwards toward your shoulders while pressing the roller. If you notice tightness then stop, take a couple of deep breaths and rock from side-to-side to release connective tissue. You can then continue to climb towards the armpit. When you are at the armpits, you can slowly move a couple of inches one side to the other to smooth away any tension in the muscles around. Repeat to the other side.

Myofascial release of hip flexors. Begin lying down on the ground using either an lacrosse ball or PVC pipe on your hip. Begin to slowly roll towards your hip and stop frequently to rock in a circular motion in order to break up the tension. When you have reached your hip, you can roll to your back and apply pressure to your TFL (tensor fasciae latae) situated between your hip and the glutes.

The final aspect is flexibility. It describes the range of motion a joint can have and also the length of muscles that connect the joints. The type of sport you're interested in will determine what amount of flexibility required. Be aware that flexibility must be considered a primary goal and something that needs to be cultivated and improved over time. If you're so tight that you cannot even touch your feet, the sport of rhythmic gymnastics may not be your ideal sport, however, just because you're naturally tight, it doesn't mean you should never try any game. This just means that extra attention must be given for a safe and enjoyable participation. Here are two exercises which can improve the flexibility of your hips as well as the shoulder.

Extend the chest and shoulders by stretching them

Begin by putting your knees and hands on the floor, with one elbow placed on the Swiss ball. Let your chest drop into the earth while reaching away from the center using your supported elbow. Consider creating a separation between your shoulder and the socket, while you hold the stretch. Maintain the posture for 45 seconds, then shake the arm for a few seconds and repeat the exercise with the opposite side.

Flexors of the hip

Take the same posture like you'd do an incline squat split, but with one knee resting upon pads for added comfort. Stretch your glutes as you slowly move your hips inward and maintain the contracting of your glutes. Keep the muscle contracting for 5 minutes. Lean the glutes back and allow the hips to drop inwards. Repeat the exercise two to three repetitions until the hips are no longer moving forward after the contraction has been released.

Try these stretching exercises every day for a few times and watch the improvement in your flexibility.

MOBILITY WORK REDUCES RISK OF INJURY FOR FIGHTERS

It's an excellent day every time an investigation is conducted that confirms your ideas as a coach of martial arts It's not just as it helps possess more information on science and also indicates that martial arts are receiving the respect they deserve. One subject area that's been much research that is long overdue, but is often ignored by both athletes and coaches is the significance of a mobility program to combat athletes. Recent research of The Journal of Strength and Conditioning was one of the first studies of its kind to take a look at the needs of injury prevention of martial arts athletes.

Researchers employed the functional movement screen (FMS) to identify limitations in balance and mobility among combatants. Although they recognized that the FMS is not well-studied in the field of martial arts, they backed the efficacy of FMS in a variety of sports. They also showed that the exercises covered in the test were similar to those that are used in martial arts.

As a martial arts instructor one of my concerns is that movement work of fighters generally is an added part of their current routines all four days a week. If the participants have done the specific martial arts exercises as well as strength and conditioning exercises prior to the training, they were told not to alter the routine. It's a great thing because it is a resemblance to the actual life of a fighter. A fightr isn't required to stop all of his activities to do mobility. The downside, however, is that a lot of fighters have a tendency to be overtraining and overtraining during the majority of their time.

The treatment proved to be effective. The study was aimed at scores higher than 14 in the FMS and also any asymmetries among the muscle groups. Scores above 14 indicate less risk of injury however, a score lower than or equal to 14 implies an 11x increased risk of injuries. Sportspersons who score of 14 or above but who also are prone to asymmetries among the muscle groups are 3x more likely to get injured.

It is clear that this will have a major consequences for combatants.

Prior to the intervention, the overall average for the of the participants was 13.25. In just four weeks, scores for the group that was undergoing intervention climbed up to 15.17 and was out of the dangerous zone. The score climbed reaching 15.33 in week 8 which showed a greater increase in the initial month.

In the event that FMS can be a reliable screen for fighters, it is apparent that symmetry and mobility (not strictly in the sense of bodybuilding) is a fantastic way for fighters to avoid injuries. In particular, the work on hips and shoulders appeared to be vital. Incorporating this exercise to the fighter's routine will improve their performances and lengthen their career.

IN DEFENSE OF SELF: THE REAL MENTAL VALUE OF SELF-DEFENSE TRAINING

Prior to discovering martial arts, I wasn't interested in joining fitness classes and preferred to be able to choose my own path and run my own way. My journey into martial arts began by taking a weekly 8-week class in the month of December. It was a challenge for me to make a commitment to an eight class program - to create my own commitment to something that I was eager to learn in order to place my interest before all else; to be there without letting other activities take precedence; and to stand up for every Monday evening from 5:30pm until 7pm, over 8 weeks. It was a battle to prove my desire to place others requirements first. I had to defend myself against putting me in a position of second importance.

The first time I began, I was receiving physical therapy to treat injuries from running. My pelvis was tipped in one direction and the other which gave me a shorter leg. It was impossible to bridge or turn towards the left to avoid my death. My body was fragile. I was overweight. It was apparent that I looked older than had. I was working to improve my fitness and had been training for an triathlon later in spring, and I was thinking that having some self-defense techniques could be useful when I was training by myself on trails.

It was an extremely difficult year. It wasn't just that I was in physical therapy and rehabilitation, but I was also in psychotherapy, too. The truth is, I didn't intend to learn physical self-defense strategies and then walk out after the eight-week program. It turns out that I was going on what we'll call "In the Defense of Self" which is a defense of fitness and health as well as of spiritual peace, of body and mind. Self that had to be rediscovered, located to be dusted off, then rebuilt.

Definition: Self-Defense

1. Protection of self in case of physical attack

2. The defense of the things that belong to oneself

The second one might be given first. It is important to understand the things that belong to you - the space you live in, your body as well as your mental or emotional state - to protect your rights. It is essential to be confident that you're worthy to protect your self-worth. It is important to recognize that it's not acceptable for people to steal away from you, whether it's something tangible such as your wallet or something intangible, such as your goals and motivation.

When I signed up for an 8-week course after each 8 weeks of training, it became something I wanted to keep. I learned how to avoid every headlock hold or wrist grabs as well as throat grasps. What do I need to know about blocking the punch or clinch how to get down, and then back up. I began to think about the best way to shift my body. I realized that I have an entire body. It wasn't my body that was an enemy. With all the time suffering from sports injuries as well as chronic sinusitis and endometriosis. doubts and discontent with my body. This did no good for me and only let me down, and even cause suffering.

Then something awe-inspiring occurred. I took my body back to be a part of the team. The hands, the arms the bridge, this bend, and I could knock someone over. I could manage my arms, my core and even the space surrounding me. The possibilities were endless - I could exercise physical control on what would take place. My body no longer an enemy, not an unending source of frustration as a trustworthy friend.

Physical Training vs. Mental Training

Physical body and the fitness training in the martial arts is only one aspect of the puzzle. Mental aspects are much more challenging to master. The physical aspect is actually much easier. You can lift this weight for 10-20 repetitions and set it up every week, and you'll notice an improvement. Change a mindset that you have relied on for fifteen twenty years, 30 years, or even longer? This is an enormous problem.

www.ingramcontent.com/pod-product-compliance
Lightning Source LLC
Chambersburg PA
CBHW070735020526
44118CB00035B/1360